NOURISH

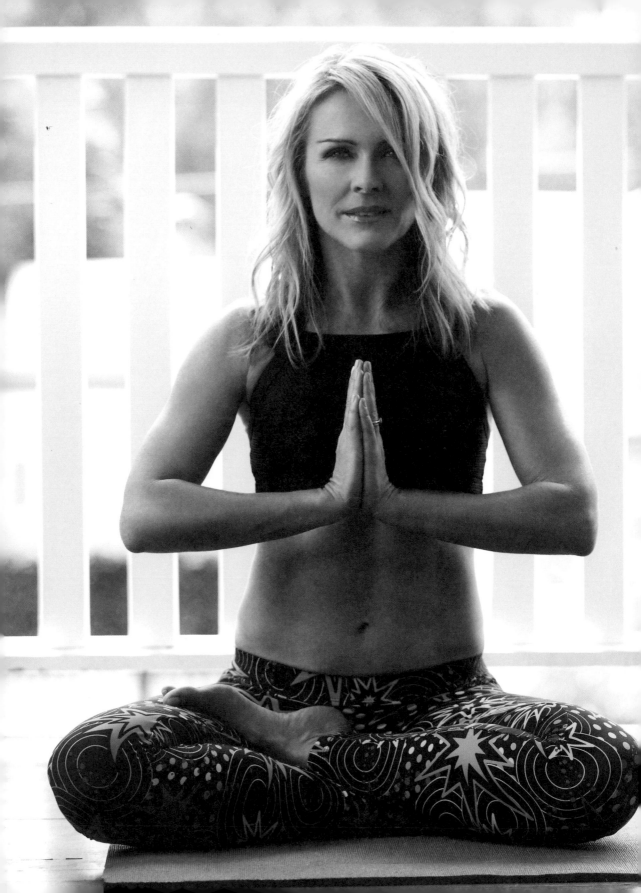

NOURISH

THE FIT WOMAN'S COOKBOOK

To Lauren
i Cathie
♡ Lorna Jane x

LORNA JANE CLARKSON

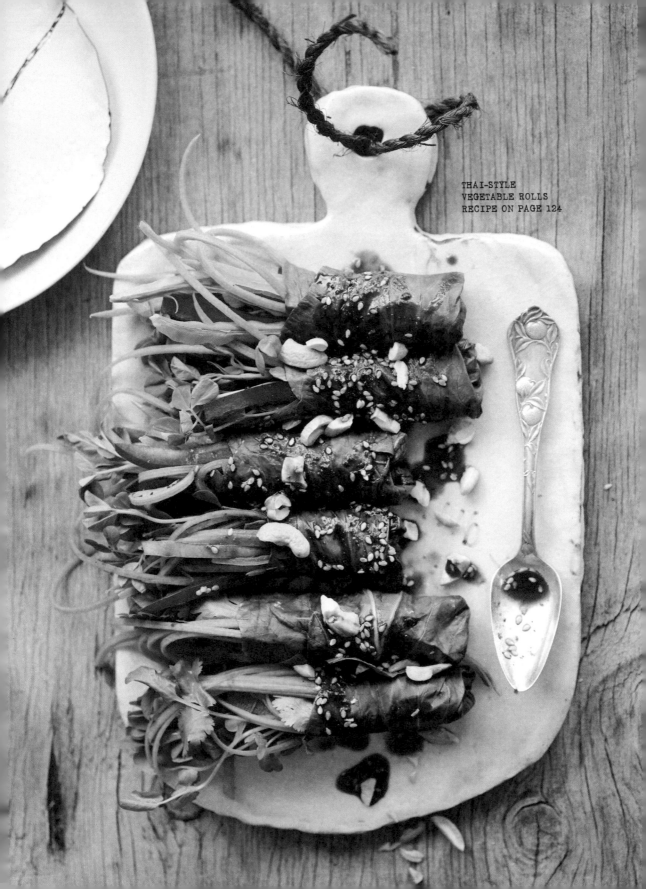

THAI-STYLE
VEGETABLE ROLLS
RECIPE ON PAGE 124

contents

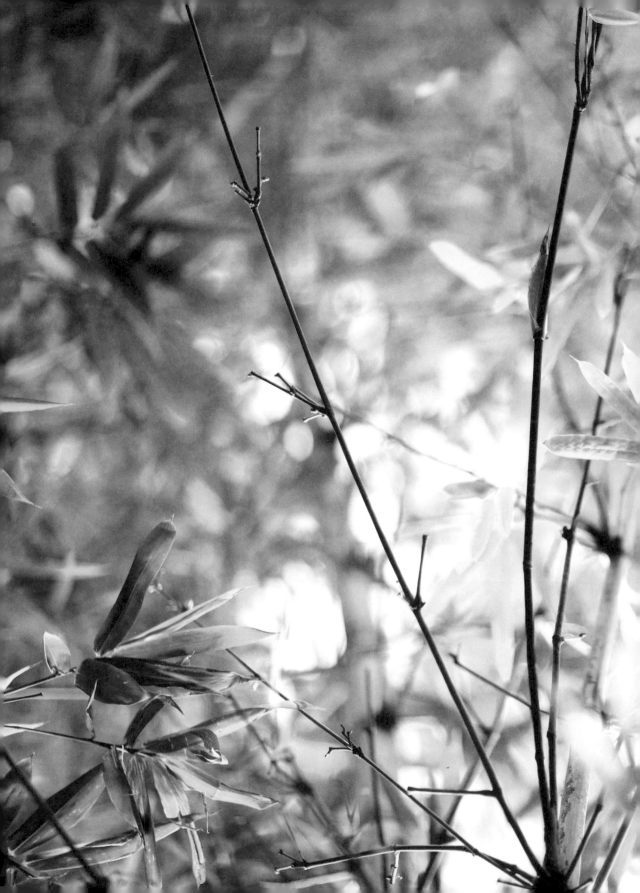

"**I BELIEVE**
THE START TO A
BETTER FUTURE
IS SIMPLY OUR BELIEF
THAT IT IS
POSSIBLE."

—— LORNA JANE CLARKSON ——

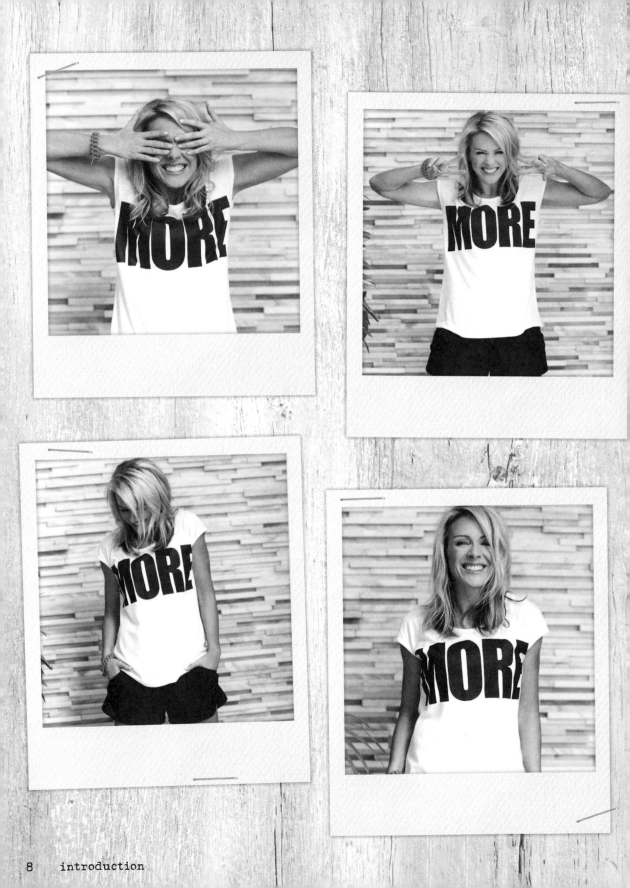

WHO IS LORNA JANE?

I am ...

Lorna Jane – a dreamer, a doer and a believer that anything is possible. I am an active wear designer, health food nut, eternal optimist and lover of all things to do with health, fitness and working out.

I choose happiness every day and I wake up knowing that great things will happen. I have a positive outlook and work to fill my life with good thoughts, good people, good health and good work.

I know my life will change me, shape me and ultimately define me. But I also know that the MORE I believe, the MORE that is possible and I am determined to make my time on this planet truly count for something by inspiring women towards

Active Living.

SO, WHAT IS ACTIVE LIVING?

Active Living is the way that I LIVE MY LIFE. It is my own personal life philosophy and one that has become a mantra for my customers and women all over the world to achieve amazing things.

Active Living: [*ak-tive; liv-ing*]
verb
1. To get more out of life by giving more of yourself every day.
2. To strive to be better each day than you were the day before.
3. To practise MOVE, NOURISH, BELIEVE
   * Moving your body every day
   * Nourishing your body with delicious food
   * Believing anything is possible if you are willing to work for it.

Active Living is about getting MORE out of life by giving MORE of yourself every day. It's a mantra that keeps me on track and full of energy despite my super-hectic schedule and it's the driving force behind everything I do. Best of all, when you break it down in to the daily practice of MOVE, NOURISH, BELIEVE – living your best, most beautiful life really isn't that hard to achieve!

I've been living this philosophy for as long as I can remember and I know first-hand how Active Living can absolutely transform lives. Every one of us has the opportunity to change for the better, to feel energised, vibrant and full of life if we just make the decision to put our health and the health of our families first – and embrace Active Living.

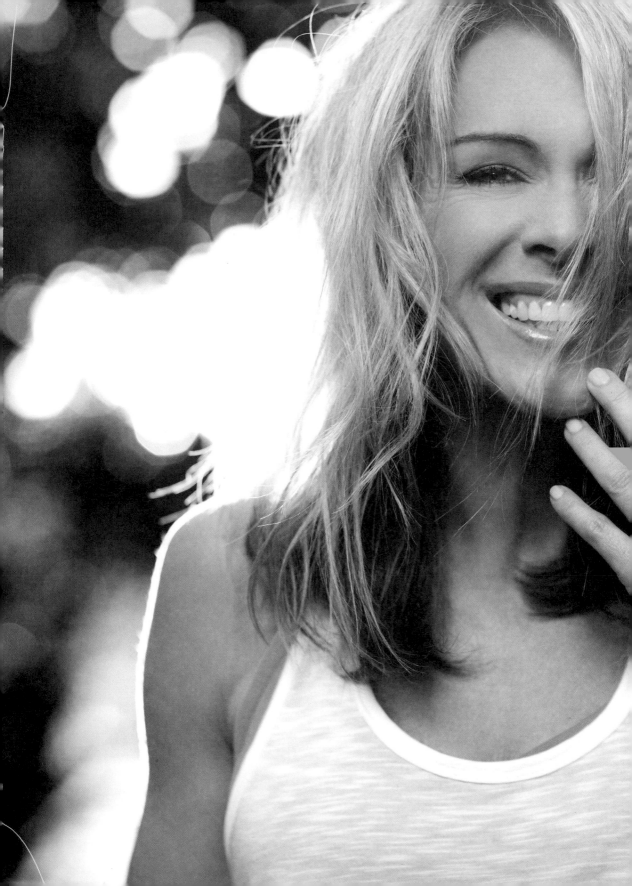

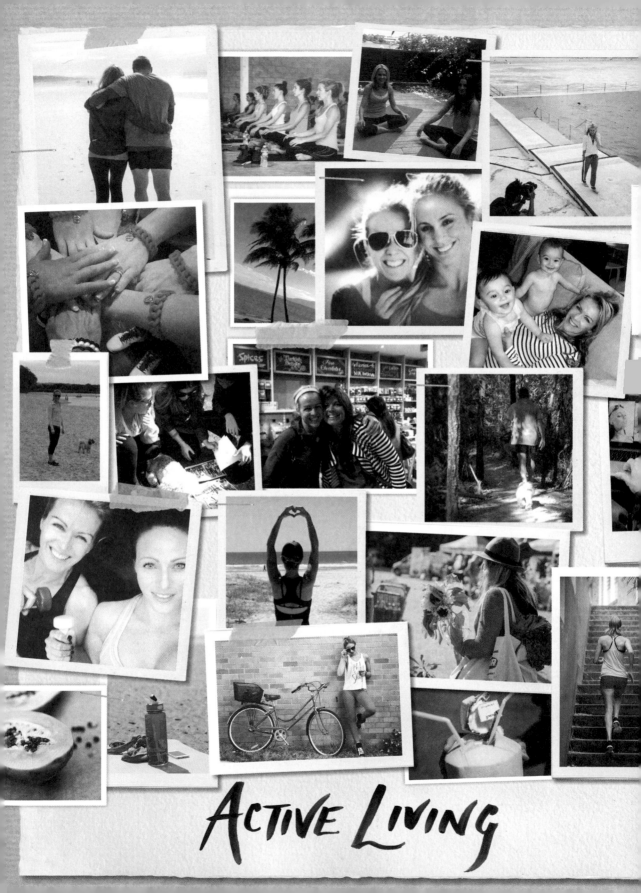

ACTIVE LIVING

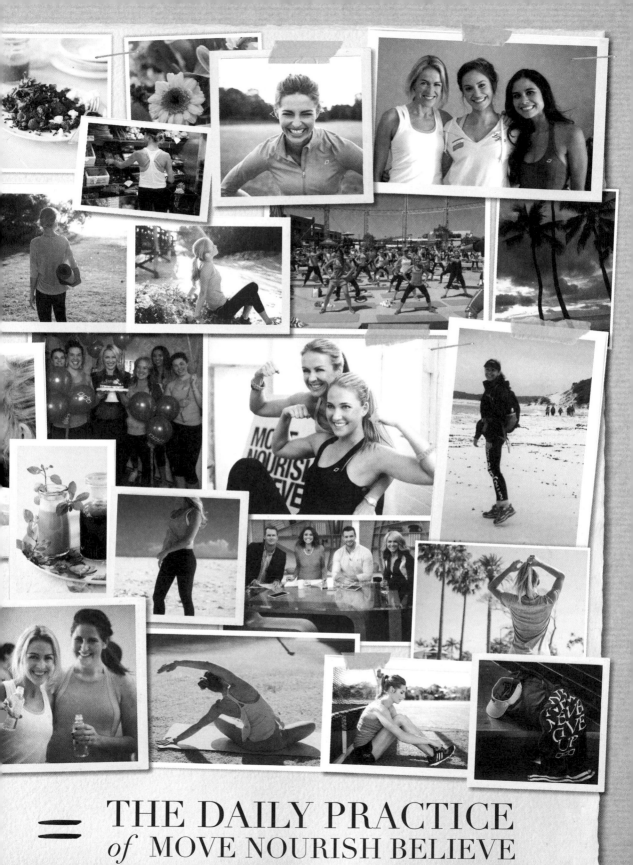

THE DAILY PRACTICE
of MOVE NOURISH BELIEVE

MY LIFE RITUALS

With the daily practice of Move Nourish Believe you can start to develop daily rituals that improve your health and wellbeing. Here are some of my life rituals that I practise every single day:

Nourish

I eat to nourish my body with whole foods that will give me the energy to live an amazing life.

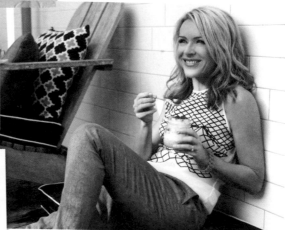

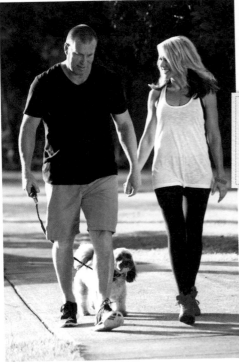

Getting outdoors

Nature offers something that simply can't be duplicated. I love to get outside a couple of times each day to re-connect and re-energise.

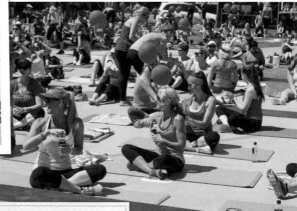

Do what you love

Be passionate about life! Always find time to do the things you love!

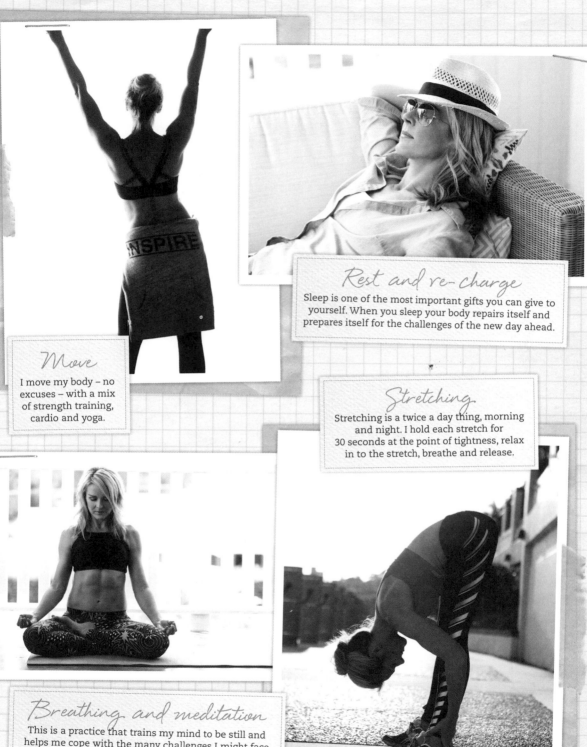

Rest and re-charge

Sleep is one of the most important gifts you can give to yourself. When you sleep your body repairs itself and prepares itself for the challenges of the new day ahead.

Move

I move my body – no excuses – with a mix of strength training, cardio and yoga.

Stretching

Stretching is a twice a day thing, morning and night. I hold each stretch for 30 seconds at the point of tightness, relax in to the stretch, breathe and release.

Breathing and meditation

This is a practice that trains my mind to be still and helps me cope with the many challenges I might face in the day-to-day running of my life and business.

you are what you eat ...

IT'S NO GREAT SECRET THAT I ADVOCATE HEALTHY EATING. I MEAN SERIOUSLY,
YOU ONLY HAVE TO SPEND A DAY IN MY LIFE TO KNOW HOW IMPORTANT
NUTRITION, FOOD AND HAVING A FIT AND HEALTHY BODY IS TO ME.

I believe the connection between what we eat and the way we look and feel is incredibly powerful. Not only does food play a vital role in supporting our health, it also defines our mental and emotional wellbeing and is a huge contributing factor to what we achieve (or don't achieve) in our lives.

So let's be honest here; it's you who decides what you eat and if I've learnt anything at all over my many years in the fitness industry, it's that you MUST take the time to think about what you eat.

I mean, REALLY take the time to stop and THINK before you reach for sugar-laden, processed or fast foods and ask: "What effect is this going to have on my health now and in the future?"

I can tell you that nutrition is not low-fat. It's not low-calorie. It's not being hungry or feeling deprived. And it's definitely not a diet that you do for six, eight or 12 weeks only to go back to your unhealthy habits as soon as you reach your 'goal weight'.

We need to NOURISH our bodies so that we can reach our full potential in life, and we need to make a commitment to do this every single day, without exception!

That is why I have written this book – I want to share my knowledge and inspire you to get off the diet treadmill, eat predominantly real foods, improve your body's digestion, hydration and alkalinity so you can look and feel better while enjoying nutritious and incredibly delicious food.

I'm talking about feeling amazing in your own skin, having a body that jumps out of bed in the morning excited about the day ahead. I'm talking about a mind that has a positive outlook, is clear and productive. And ultimately, I'm talking about living your best, most rewarding and fun-filled life.

This book is a collection of all of the things I have learned and love about nourishing my body. It is a representation of my food philosophies, of what I think about when I'm choosing ingredients, how I balance nutritional content and an insight in to the foods I choose to eat and why.

I really hope you enjoy my favourite recipes and that you are inspired to think before you eat, make good decisions and truly give your body the nourishment it deserves.

> **IF YOU HONESTLY WANT TO TAKE CARE OF YOURSELF BOTH PHYSICALLY AND MENTALLY YOU NEED TO STOP AND TAKE CARE OF THE WAY YOU FEED YOURSELF FIRST.**

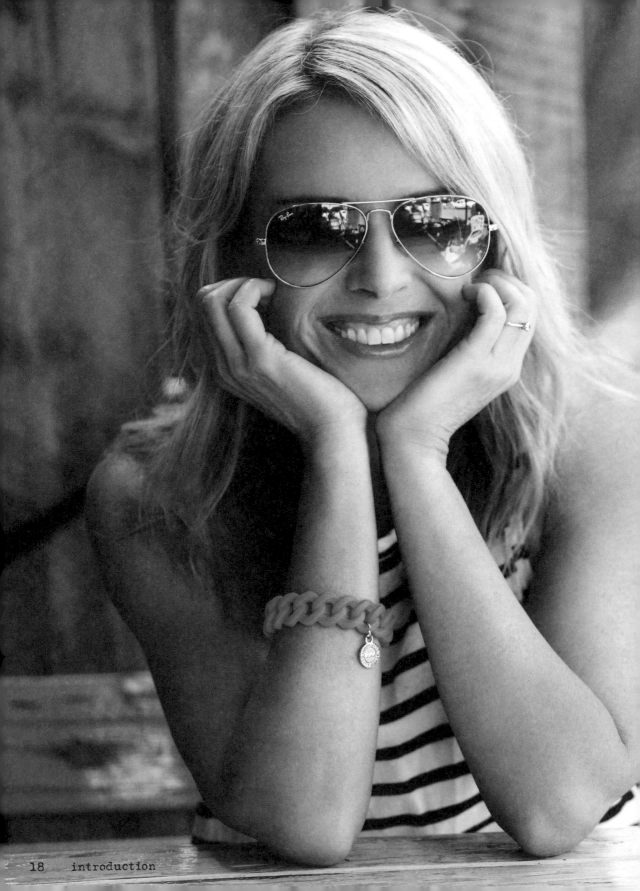

"SO...
LET'S BE HONEST HERE;
IT'S YOU
WHO DECIDES WHAT
YOU EAT!"

STOP DIETING!

Okay, so I admit I'm a little frustrated by the culture of dieting that we have in our society. It just seems like we are confronted with it at every level – on TV shows, in magazines, in movies...

Even on a personal level, we all have at least one person in our lives who is constantly on a new diet, or talking about a diet or trying to get you to go on a diet with them. It just seems like we have accepted it as a way of life.

Well, I'm here to tell you that you don't have to diet! In fact, I believe it is one of the worst things you can do for your mental and physical health not to mention your metabolism, mood and social life.

The simple truth is that diets just don't work and we need to make a promise not to deny or deprive ourselves when it comes to food. We need to make a commitment to love and nourish our bodies and give them what they need to be healthy, fit and strong.

Eating is all about balance and when you get it right you won't feel hungry or deprived, and you won't be compromising your health and wellbeing either.

IN A NUTSHELL, DIETS JUST DON'T WORK AND HERE'S WHY:

✱ The weight lost is too fast.

✱ They destroy a healthy metabolism and make it even more difficult for our bodies to look and feel at their best. And that's before we start thinking about fighting disease, ageing and keeping our hair, skin and nails looking good.

✱ They can cause illness, as you are not meeting all your nutritional needs.

✱ They become addictive and you end up on an endless treadmill of yo-yo dieting. When one doesn't work, you try another, and then another and it doesn't stop!

✱ They are harmful to your self-esteem. As most diets are destined to fail due to the extreme deprivation that is their nature, you end up feeling guilty and ashamed.

✱ They don't take in to account that we are all individuals and as such have different energy outputs, so require different food and quantities of foods to meet our specific needs.

✱ Diets do not allow you to function normally. If you constantly have to measure, count, restrict and obsess over food, you feel punished, deprived, even angry. And that's no way to live your life!

REALITY CHECK!

YOU ARE THE DRIVER OF YOUR OWN LIFE SO DON'T LET FAD DIETS RULE WHO YOU ARE! MAKE A PROMISE TO YOURSELF TO STOP COUNTING CALORIES AND FOCUS ON FEEDING YOUR BODY THE HEALTH-PROMOTING NUTRIENTS IT NEEDS TO BE POWERFUL AND STRONG!

Stop Dieting!
Stop Dieting!
Oh, and did
I mention
Stop Dieting!

> I DON'T HAVE A STRICT RULE ABOUT HOW MANY MEALS AND SNACKS I EAT EACH DAY, BUT I DO LISTEN TO MY BODY AND GIVE IT WHAT IT NEEDS TO FEEL GREAT.

CARAWAY BEETROOT DIP
RECIPE ON PAGE 148

DETOX GREEN SOUP
RECIPE ON PAGE 100

detox soup

dEtox soup

EAT LESS, MORE OFTEN

I've spoken about the importance of not dieting. So now I want to talk about how important it is to listen to your body's needs when it comes to food, to eat smaller portions more frequently and,most importantly, not to SKIP MEALS.

When you skip meals, or leave several hours between each meal, your metabolism slows down and you stop burning calories at the rate you should. Then because you have stopped feeding it, your body thinks you're starving, so it begins to conserve energy and store food, usually as fat! Subsequently, when you finally decide to eat again, your body naturally wants to store fat just in case you forget to eat again! So if you don't want to become a 'fat-storing machine' don't skip meals!

SKIPPING MEALS IS A BAD IDEA

But the good news is that when you start to eat smaller meals more frequently, and especially when you include metabolism-boosting fresh fruit and vegetables, your body will use this fuel at a higher rate (which boosts your metabolism). And it will stop storing it as fat, because it knows you will be eating again soon.

I don't have a strict rule about how many meals and snacks I eat each day but I do try to listen to my body and eat when it tells me to. I want to make sure that I give myself enough energy and nutrition to be at my best every day and I find the key to getting this right is planning ahead and developing rituals that work for me and what I have planned for the day.

HOW I MAKE EATING LESS, MORE OFTEN WORK FOR ME:

✳ What I eat for breakfast and when depends on what I have planned for my morning and how hungry I am from the night before. If my plan is to do yoga I will just have some fruit and my energy tonic (for recipe, see page 42), but if I am strength training with my trainer, I will have something more substantial like a smoothie or some soaked oats (page 57).

✳ After training if I'm feeling super hungry I will have a frittata (page 132) or some smashed eggs on toast (page 68), otherwise I will whip up a smoothie with some protein in it (page 95) and take it to work with me.

✳ Lunch is usually a salad with protein or a soup with a salad in the cooler months. If I'm working out in the afternoon or I know dinner will be late, I have a snack around 4pm. I choose something easy to digest, but I'm always sure to have a few options on-hand so I am not tempted to raid the vending machine at work!

✳ Dinner is most often at home and I try not to eat too late, so my body has enough time to digest it before I sleep. If I feel like it, I have dessert, but I allow a little time after my meal so I don't overload my digestive system. I also find that I enjoy it more if I wait a little too.

My philosophy with food is about eating according to what you feel your body needs for the day ahead – not being greedy, but not depriving yourself either. Think about the day ahead, listen to your body and give yourself the nourishment you need to be at your best.

LOOK GOOD, FEEL GREAT

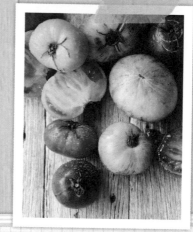

THE BEST strategy to look and feel at your best is to banish processed and refined foods from your life and eat a predominantly REAL food diet. That is, bucket loads of fresh fruit and vegetables, a variety of whole grains, the right kinds of proteins and fats and, of course, plenty of water.

The definition of REAL food is pretty straightforward. It's food grown or raised with few or no chemicals, hormones, sprays or other weird bioengineering tactics or processing – like the food you would grow in your own backyard.

Real food is food you recognise, that your kids should recognise and that your parents and grandparents were raised on. It comes from plants or from animals and doesn't have to pass through a factory or chemistry lab to land on your plate.

So let's start with the most important nutrition-delivering ingredients of them all: **FRUIT and VEGETABLES.**

Making fruit and vegetables your new best friends is one of the most rewarding things you will ever do for your body. They're packed full of essential vitamins, minerals and antioxidants and will have you looking and feeling wonderful in no time at all.

MY SUPERSTAR FRUIT AND VEGETABLES

GREEN LEAFY VEGETABLES
These should be part of your routine, every day, so include them in your smoothies and salads – no excuses! I mix it up but my absolute faves are broccoli and spinach, because they cleanse the liver to keep my blood flowing and skin glowing. They also contain coenzyme Q10, which is a powerful antioxidant.

TOMATOES
Aside from tasting great, tomatoes contain lycopene, a powerful antioxidant and anti-cancer agent. And did you know that cooking tomatoes increases the lycopene by more than five times? It's true! Include them in your sauces, frittatas and soups, or roast some in coconut oil and add to your salads!

BERRIES
Berries are my anti-ageing heroes. They're packed with vitamin C and antioxidants. I sprinkle a few over my cereal in the morning, toss them into my smoothies or enjoy them on their own as a dessert.

REAL FOODS are what humans are meant to eat for optimal health and nutrition and an all-important part of that is wholegrains, proteins and good fats.

Wholegrains are nature's comfort foods and if you peek into my pantry you'll find a wide variety of containers filled with not just brown rice, but purple and black rice too. There are also tubs of quinoa, mixed, black and white, as well as an array of breakfast cereals ranging from gluten-free whole oats to homemade natural muesli, granola, and chia. I love to include these in my recipes and buy most of them from my local health food store or market. I buy them mostly from the 'serve yourself' containers and then store them in glass jars once I get home.

I also have what some would call a slight addiction to superfoods such as goji berries, acai, dried blueberries, coconut flakes and bee pollen (to name a few) and I store these alongside my grains in easy reach for a quick snack or as a topping for my next smoothie.

I want to be as strong and healthy as possible, so I make sure that I eat protein often and from a wide variety of sources.

MY GO-TO FAVOURITES ARE:

* White fish
* Free-range, organic chicken breast
* Free-range, cruelty-free, organic whole eggs
* Prawns
* Protein powder

I also know that the best way to eat protein is in small portions throughout the day, making it easier on my digestive system and to ensure the amino acids are constantly available for my body to build and repair.

Fats have had a bad rap in the past, but knowing the fats that are good for your body is essential. Good fats keep your hunger at bay and help to maintain beautiful, youthful-looking skin. Omega 3 fats are the best for our skin and filling up on foods containing them, such as salmon and walnuts, is a great way to fight wrinkles and stay looking younger for longer.

THE FATS I ALWAYS HAVE IN MY KITCHEN ARE:

* Certified organic extra-virgin coconut oil
* Extra-virgin olive oil
* Salmon (which I eat once or twice a week)
* A wide variety of nuts and seeds
* Avocados

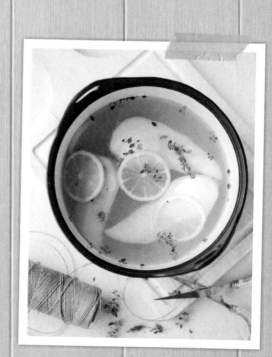

POACHED CHICKEN
RECIPE ON PAGE 245

WHERE DO I SHOP?

I always buy local and in season because I find locally-grown foods are always fresher, taste better and usually less expensive too. The cornerstone of my food shopping is a weekly trip to the local farmer's market to discover the best quality produce possible and I plan my meals for the week ahead from the very best the season has to offer.

I love the atmosphere of my local market and always make time to talk to the growers. I find their passion for food infectious and they'll often share fantastic advice about anything from how to select the juiciest citrus fruit, through to clever storage tips and often some great recipe ideas too.

Throughout the week, I head to my local greengrocer or health food store to pick up fresh supplies. Although it may cost a few dollars more than the big supermarkets, I view the food I eat as an investment in my future health and wellbeing and when you consider how much money can easily be wasted on poor quality produce it's well and truly worthwhile.

I buy my meat from a local, ethical butcher and always look for grass-fed, pasture-raised organic beef. I buy only ethical organic free-range eggs and poultry and I visit a local fishmonger for my fish and seafood and choose only wild and not farmed.

I believe the quality of our food is paramount for good health and there is something inherently wrong with eating foods out of season. They may have been frozen, imported or kept in storage for a long time, all the while diminishing in taste and nutrients. Bottom-line ... low in nutrition and just not good for you.

When organic produce is not readily available a quick and easy way to remove some of the pesticides from your fruit and vegetables is to mix up one tablespoon of apple cider vinegar with one cup of water. Place your produce in the solution and leave for five minutes, stirring now and then. Remove the produce, rinse well and dry. (Only soak the produce you plan on using that day.) Another quick and easy way to do this is to put the mixture in a spray bottle and spray your produce and rinse and dry as you go.

HOW IMPORTANT IS ORGANIC?

When I shop I try to buy organic whenever I can but honestly, it is more important to me that the produce is fresh, in season and locally grown. You can tell just by looking, smelling and touching the produce whether it's good for you – you don't need an organic label to tell you that!

When you ARE shopping for 'organic' watch for labelling. If food has been certified by a leading body, such as Australian Certified Organic, or in the USA an accredited agent that falls under the banner of USDA Certified Organic, then (and only then) can you be sure it's truly organic.

But remember – organic doesn't always mean REAL foods either! So watch that your organic food doesn't look too overly processed or refined.

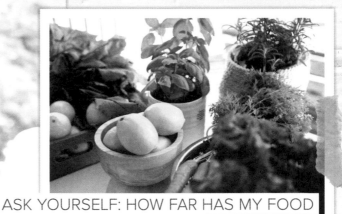

"ASK YOURSELF: HOW FAR HAS MY FOOD TRAVELLED TO GET TO MY PLATE? WHAT IS THE ENVIRONMENTAL IMPACT OF THAT JOURNEY? HAS IT BEEN TREATED WITH CHEMICALS? REMEMBER, THE CLOSER TO HOME THE SOURCE, THE BETTER FOR YOU, YOUR COMMUNITY AND THE PLANET."

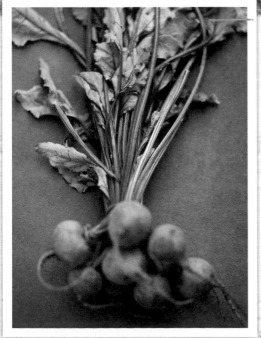

MEXICAN FISH AND QUINOA
SALAD RECIPE ON PAGE 110

seasonal eating

> Choosing fruit and vegetables in season means you are eating food that has been grown and harvested in peak conditions.

VEGETABLES

spring

artichokes, globe
asian greens
asparagus
avocados
beans, broad (fava); green
beetroot (beets)
broccoli
carrots
cauliflower
chillies
corn
cucumber
garlic
lettuce
mushrooms
onions, green (scallions); spring
peas
potatoes
silver beet (swiss chard)
spinach
tomatoes
watercress
zucchini
zucchini flowers

summer

asparagus
avocados
beans, butter; green; flat; snake
capsicum (bell pepper)
celery
chillies
choko (chayote)
corn
cucumber
eggplant
lettuce
okra
onions, green (scallions); spring
peas, sugar snap
potatoes
radish
squash
tomatoes
watercress
zucchini

autumn

asian greens
avocados
beans
broccoli
brussels sprouts
cabbage
capsicum (bell pepper)
carrots
cauliflower
celery
celeriac (celery root)
chestnuts
choko (chayote)
corn
cucumber
eggplant
fennel
ginger
kumara (orange sweet potato)
leek
lettuce
mushrooms
okra
onions
parsnip
potatoes
pumpkin
shallots
silver beet (swiss chard)
spinach
tomatoes
turnips
witlof (belgian endive)
zucchini

winter

avocados
beetroot (beets)
broccoli
brussels sprouts
cabbage
carrots
cauliflower
celeriac (celery root)
celery
fennel
jerusalem artichokes (sunchokes)
kohlrabi
kumara (orange sweet potato)
leek
okra
olives
onions
parsnip
potatoes
pumpkin
silver beet (swiss chard)
spinach
swede
turnips
witlof (belgian endive)

FRUIT

spring

apples

bananas

berries – blueberries, mulberries, strawberries

cherries

grapefruit

lemons

loquats

mandarins, honey murcot

mangoes

oranges, blood; seville; valencia

passionfruit

papaya; pawpaw

pineapple

pomelo

rockmelon

tangelos

summer

apricots

bananas

berries – blackberries, blueberries, currants (red & white), raspberries, strawberries

cherries

figs

grapes

limes

lychees

mangoes

mangosteens

melons

nectarines

oranges, valencia

passionfruit

peaches

pears, williams; howell

pineapple

plums

rambutans

autumn

apples

bananas

custard apples

figs

guava

kiwifruit

lemons

limes

mandarins, imperial

mangosteens

nashi

oranges, valencia; navel

passionfruit

pawpaw

pears

persimmons

plums

pomegranates

quince

rhubarb

tamarillo

winter

apples

bananas

berries – strawberries

cumquats

custard apples

grapefruit

kiwifruit

lemons

mandarins

nashi

oranges, navel; blood

passionfruit, panama

pears

pomelo

quince

rhubarb

tangelos

Buy local, buy in season and support your local community and your body's nutritional requirements all at the same time!

LET'S TALK ABOUT HYDRATION

Water is the number one essential ingredient for good health and the cheapest anti-ageing potion on the planet! Every cell, tissue and organ in our bodies needs water to function and the more fresh and clean water we consume, the more efficiently every process in our bodies is going to operate.

Our bodies use water to maintain temperature, digest food, cleanse cells and eliminate waste. And drinking water gives us:

* More energy
* Better digestion
* A higher metabolism
* Fewer cravings
* Fewer headaches
* A better mood and outlook
* The ability to concentrate more
* Better weight management
* More efficient toxin removal
* Clear, glowing skin
* Less fatigue
* Improved overall health and wellbeing

Starting the day with water is essential and I like to drink a litre of water as soon as I wake up. If I follow this simple morning ritual it makes me want to sip water all day.

I always have a bottle of water by my side which I drink at room temperature to increase absorption. I also avoid drinking water with meals as too much liquid can dilute digestive juices which slows digestion and can cause bloating and discomfort.

If you find it difficult to drink just plain water, add sliced cucumber, fresh berries, apple, mint or lemon to infuse natural flavour and goodness into the mix. Think of it as nature's cordial. Other ways to increase your water intake are by drinking caffeine-free herbal tea (see page 228), or in the wintertime, in a nourishing vegetable soup.

If you're new to this, set yourself realistic goals. Aim to have a glass of water when you wake, one half an hour before each meal and snack, and one again before you go to bed. Eventually, you will become so accustomed to drinking water that it will feel strange not to have it with you at all times.

Remember, there are times when you need to increase your water intake. This includes when you're exercising, if you're in a sauna or steam room and after having a massage.

HOW MUCH TO DRINK?

It's recommended that we drink between two and three litres of water each day (or eight glasses). Drinking water at certain times of the day helps maximise its effectiveness. Here is a quick guide:

✻ Two glasses after waking helps activate internal organs.
✻ One glass 30 minutes before eating aids digestion.
✻ One glass before taking a shower or bath helps lower blood pressure.

GOOD DIGESTION = GOOD HEALTH

Your digestive system is the epicentre of your health.

It's where your body extracts its nutrients and it is an integral part of your body's immune defence system. The healthier your digestive system, the better it can process food, break nutrients down and absorb all of the good stuff your cells need every day.

We all know it's essential that we feed our bodies with fresh, nutrient-dense foods, but if our digestive system is not operating efficiently, we won't receive the nutrients we need from our food to function at our best.

So here are a few tips you can follow to make sure you're digesting your food correctly and receiving all of the delicious nutrients your body deserves.

✳ Sit down and eat mindfully. A rushed meal encourages poor protein metabolism, bloating and bad digestion.

✳ Don't drink while you are eating a meal. Drinking too much during mealtimes can dilute digestive juices and slow down the digestive process.

✳ Chew slowly. Chew each mouthful at least 20 times before swallowing to ensure each mouthful is pre-digested by the enzyme ptyalin, found in your saliva. If you can do this (or at least chew each mouthful a little more than usual), your stomach won't have to work as hard and the absorption of important vitamins and nutrients will occur more efficiently.

✳ Look after your gut health. It is essential that you have the correct amount of good and bad bacteria in your gut for optimum digestion. To help preserve the correct balance and a healthy digestive environment, I recommend you include a probiotic in to your daily routine. You can find these in yoghurt or take them as a powdered supplement in your smoothies or in capsule form from your local naturopath.

✳ Last but not least, an age-old digestive remedy, apple cider vinegar, is great for promoting optimal digestion and encourages the growth of friendly bacteria in your body. Look for one that is 'raw' or 'unfiltered' and either drink it before your evening meal (one tablespoon diluted in a cup of water) or simply add it as part of the dressing on a salad. It is high in minerals and potassium and has antiseptic qualities that help cleanse your digestive system.

The healthier your digestive system, the better it can process food and absorb all the good stuff.

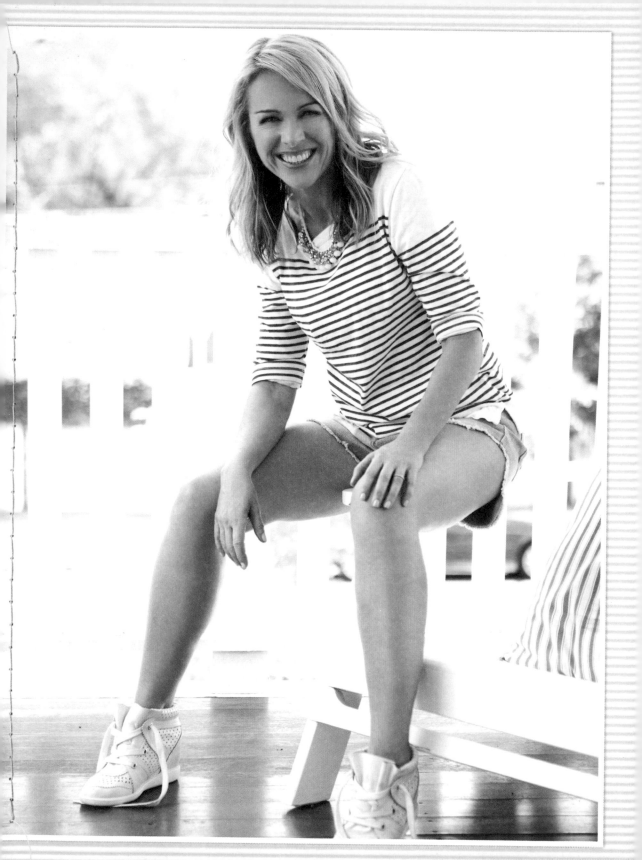

ALKALINITY

The acid/alkaline level of your body (known as the pH level) is important for the health of all of your cells and tissues. Keeping your body in an alkaline state will also improve your mood, energy levels and sleep quality. Not to mention reducing aches and pains, headaches and chronic disease.

The foods we eat can affect how acidic or alkaline we become. Some foods break down into acid-forming substances, where others assist in keeping our bodies at their health-promoting alkaline-best.

The key is balance and ideally, your diet should be made up of 80 per cent alkaline-forming foods and 20 per cent acid-forming foods.

And guess what? It is not only the foods we eat that affect our body's alkalinity. Strenuous exercise can also make the body more acidic by making your blood acidic. So, if you tend to push yourself to the limit in cardio or weights, try to balance it out with gentle exercises like yoga, tai chi and chi gong. They gently stimulate your lymph to remove acid waste from the body that can build up after a hardcore workout.

Deep breathing also makes the blood more alkaline, so be sure to practise a little meditation every day.

ACIDIC FOODS INCLUDE:
* Sugar
* Meat (including pork)
* Fish
* Poultry
* Eggs
* Cheese
* Bread
* Rice
* Oats
* Processed food
* Refined products
* Alcohol
* Caffeine

ALKALINE FOODS INCLUDE:
* Most fresh fruit
* Green vegetables (asparagus, broccoli, spinach, etc)
* Peas
* Beans
* Lentils
* Herbs and seasonings
* Seeds and nuts
* Seaweed
* Spirulina
* Water
* Onion
* Pineapple
* Sweet potato
* Watermelon

> **EATING MORE ALKALINE FOODS PROMOTES BETTER HEALTH AND OVERALL WELLBEING.**

LET'S TALK ABOUT HOW TO TEST YOUR PH AND WHAT IS THE NORMAL ZONE:

The balance between alkalinity and acidity is referred to as our PH level. And it ranges from being totally acidic (zero pH) to totally alkaline (14pH) with 7pH being neutral – and where we want our bodies to be. By balancing the amounts of acid-forming and alkaline-forming food we eat, we can achieve a body that is more alkaline and as a result healthier and more youthful.

enjoyment!

Enjoyment is my number one consideration when deciding what to eat. But I also want my food to have the nutrients to fuel a mind and body that I'm proud of, that is full of health and capability and that allows me to achieve all of the things I have to do each and every day.

So what I look for is food that can give my body everything it needs nutritionally, while also being delicious and satisfying enough to keep my tastebuds happy at the same time. I also want food and recipes that I can enjoy with my family and friends without having to apologise for the taste or keep having to tell them to eat it 'because it's good for them!'

Food is meant to be enjoyed and one of the common misconceptions about healthy food is that it doesn't have the enjoyment-factor of fast, fried, flavour-enhanced or sugar-laden 'fun foods'.

But believe me when I tell you (and show you with the recipes in this book) that this is not the case. You absolutely can have enjoyment, deliciousness and healthiness in the foods you eat – all at the same time.

It frustrates me that so many people spend their entire lives not knowing how great they can look and feel, or how clear their minds can be because they eat overly processed, anti-nutrient foods. I want to shout it from the roof-tops that no matter how old or young or unfit and unhealthy you are it is never too late – you can turn your health around right now by eating good food today.

One of the easiest and most important things to do when ridding your life of unhealthy foods is to replace some of the 'naughty' foods you regularly enjoy and look forward to with healthier alternatives.

It could be as simple as swapping a whip-cream topped hot chocolate for a more nutritious (and more tasty) chai tea or chai latte. Or swapping your favourite chocolate bar for some homemade cacao truffles. Or even swapping your regular morning bottled orange juice for a freshly squeezed and full of goodness one you made for yourself.

Start by making a list of all the foods you currently enjoy, work out the ones that are detrimental to your health and then find some alternatives that you can enjoy instead. It may take some adjustment but trust me, you will start to look forward to and enjoy these healthier alternatives in as little as a few days.

Healthy habits are just as addictive as unhealthy ones. Just make small changes every day and before you know it, you'll be on the road to better nutrition and better health while enjoying guilt-free foods at the same time.

Go ahead, get started and begin to enjoy better food, a better more capable body and an altogether better YOU!

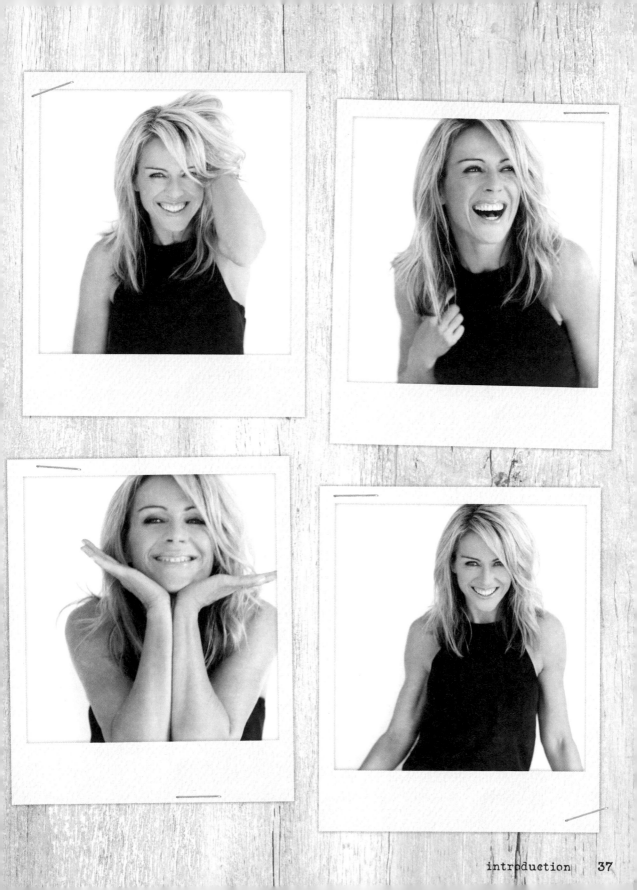

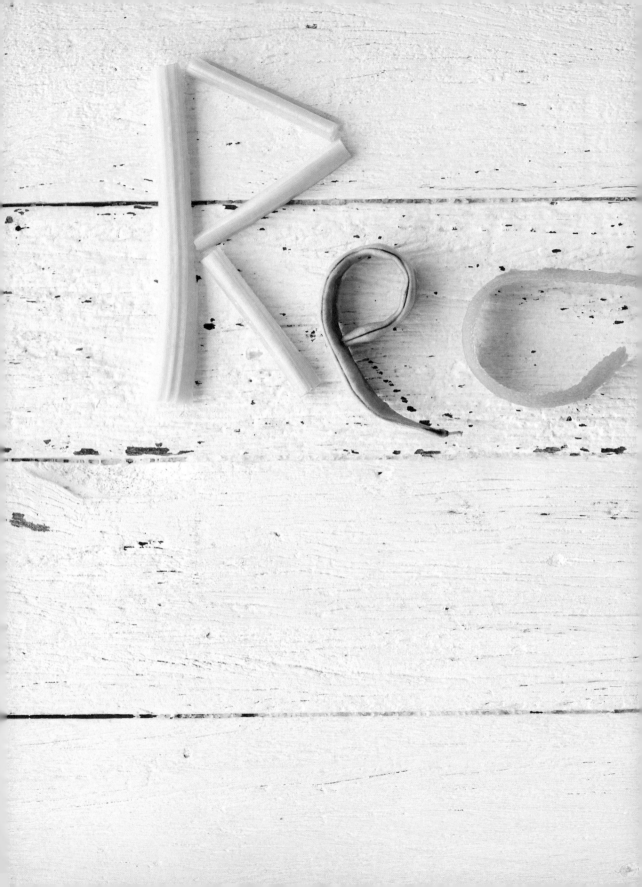

We've talked about the importance of **ACTIVE LIVING** and the daily practice of **MOVE NOURISH BELIEVE**. I've given you insights into what I think you should consider when you're deciding how to nourish your body. So now it's time to share with you some of my fave guilt-free, nutritious and delicious recipes.

The following recipes are ones that are made in my kitchen almost every week. They are easy enough to prepare when you have a busy schedule and so delicious you will want to enjoy them over and over again.

You will notice that most of the ingredients can be used in a number of recipes so they won't sit unused in your pantry and I have also designed the recipes so you can easily adjust them to suit any amazing in-season produce that you find at your local farmer's market.

I hope you LOVE what you are about to discover and that you'll be inspired to share your favourites with your friends and encourage and inspire the people in your life towards Active Living and a healthier, more nutritious approach to eating.

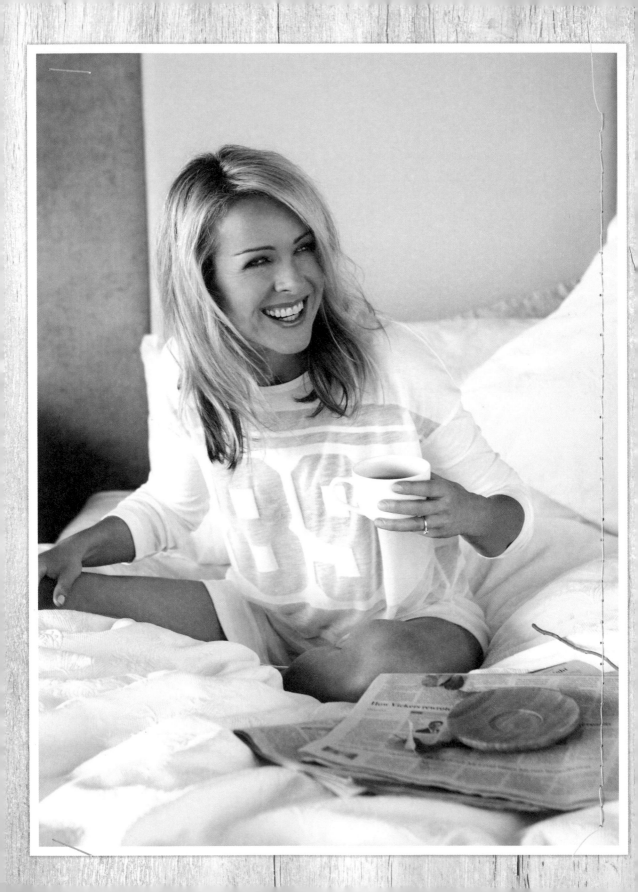

WAKE UP

I love a good health retreat! And something I've discovered over years of escaping to one retreat or another, is the many health benefits of tonics and elixirs. Simply put, they are a concentrate of highly potent ingredients, in health-promoting combinations designed to give you an instant boost of whatever your body needs on a particular day.

There are nine in this book and you will find one for energy, one for immunity, one for happiness and even one to boost your metabolism. I usually make one first thing in the morning and customise it to suit what I need for that particular day. I quite often make a double batch and save one for the afternoon so I can get an extra dose of whatever I need.

I am constantly amazed at the power of nutrient-rich foods and have made these powerful doses of goodness an essential part of my day.

energy TONIC

Combine 2 x 30ml (1 ounce) espresso coffee shots, ⅓ cup (80ml) boiling water, 2 teaspoons coconut sugar, 1 tablespoon cacao powder and a pinch of cayenne pepper in a small heatproof jug until coffee and sugar are dissolved. Pour into serving glasses or bottles.

----

prep time 5 minutes
serves 2 (about 75ml each)
nutritional count per serving protein (1.1g), carbohydrate (3.2g), total fat (0.5g), fibre (0g).

I limit myself to one coffee a day and try not to have any caffeine after lunch. I do this to make sure I can relax and unwind towards the end of the day and sleep well through the night.

cook's notes

For chilled juices, use refrigerated ingredients.

Coconut sugar and cacao powder are available from health food stores.

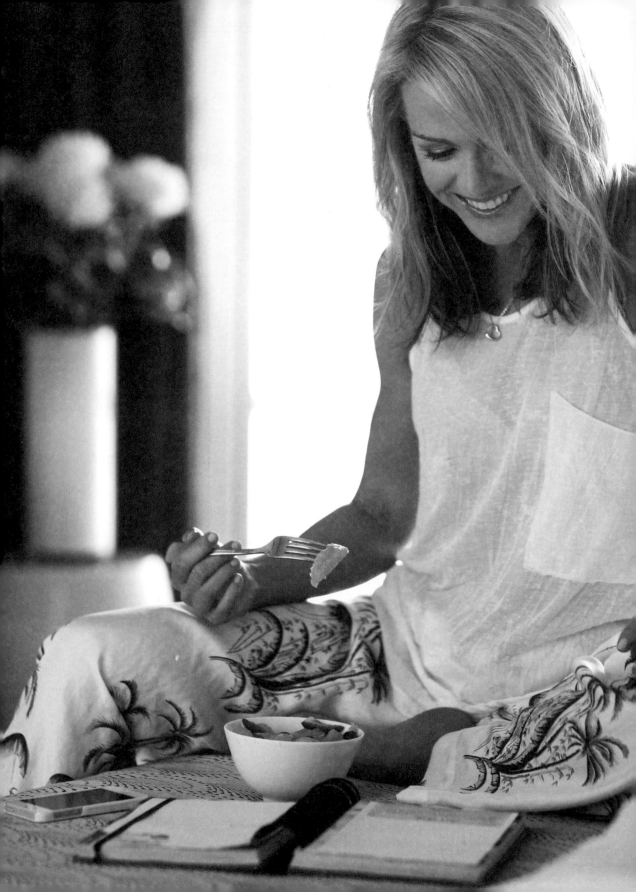

"**NUTRITION IS THE KEY** TO OVERALL GOOD HEALTH AND **PROPER NUTRITION** IS ESSENTIAL FOR US TO LOOK, THINK AND PERFORM **AT OUR BEST.**"

immunity TONIC

Whisk ½ cup (125ml) freshly squeezed orange juice with grated 1cm (½-inch) piece fresh ginger, 2 teaspoons manuka honey and grated 1cm (½-inch) piece fresh turmeric in a small jug until combined. Pour into serving glasses or bottles.

----

prep time 5 minutes
serves 2 (about 75ml each)
nutritional count per serving protein (0.4g), carbohydrate (10.7g), total fat (0.1g), fibre (0.2g).

cook's notes

If you can't find fresh turmeric, you can use a pinch of ground turmeric instead. Always wear plastic kitchen gloves when handling turmeric as it will stain your hands.

Manuka honey is known to have antibacterial and antiviral properties and has been found to be effective against sore throats, stomach ulcers and skin infections. It also contains antioxidants which increase immunity.

----

happiness TONIC

Whisk ½ cup (125ml) pure coconut water with grated 1cm (½-inch) piece fresh turmeric, 2 teaspoons manuka honey and ¼ teaspoon ground cinnamon in a small jug until combined. Pour into serving glasses or bottles. Sprinkle with some bee pollen on top before serving, if you like.

----

prep time 5 minutes
serves 2 (about 75ml each)
nutritional count per serving protein (0.3g), carbohydrate (9g), total fat (0.1g), fibre (0g).

beauty TONIC

Mash ½ cup (100g) thawed frozen mixed berries in a small bowl with a fork. Stir in ¼ cup (60ml) freshly squeezed orange juice and 1 tablespoon white chia seeds. Pour mixture into serving glasses or bottles. Stand 30 minutes or until thickened before serving.

----

prep time 5 minutes (+ standing)
serves 2 (about 75ml each)
nutritional count per serving protein (1.9g), carbohydrate (6.6g), total fat (3.1g), fibre (2g).

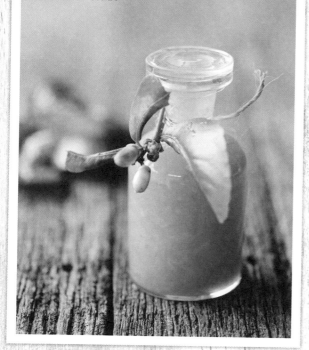

IMMUNITY TONIC

cook's notes

We used pure coconut water from a fresh, young coconut. When buying packaged coconut water, avoid those with added sweeteners or preservatives.

Bee pollen is both medicinal and delicious. With its intense honey burst and crunch, it is also rich in proteins, free amino acids, vitamins (including B-complex) and folic acid. It also contains antibiotic factors and is thought to help improve immunity and vitality.

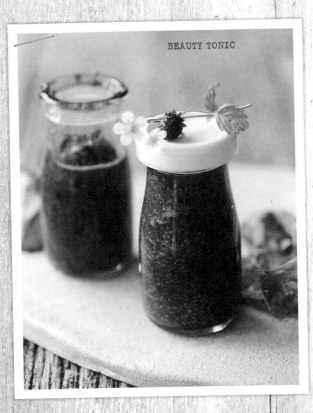

BEAUTY TONIC

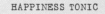

HAPPINESS TONIC

I recommend coconut water as a good, natural option to replenish electrolytes, but be sure to stick to natural, unsweetened brands only.

metabolism-booster ELIXIR

Peel and coarsely chop ¼ small pineapple (225g). Push pineapple, 0.5cm (¼-inch) piece fresh ginger (5g) and ½ bunch fresh mint through a juice extractor into a small jug. Stir in 2 tablespoons coconut water. Pour into serving glasses or bottles. Serve sprinkled with a pinch of cayenne pepper.

----

prep time 5 minutes
serves 2 (about 80ml each)
nutritional count per serving protein (0.2g), carbohydrate (8.6g), total fat (0.2g), fibre (2g).

cook's notes

We used pure coconut water from a fresh young drinking coconut. To check the freshness of a young coconut, press your finger into the centre of the base. If it is firm, then the coconut is fresh. If peeled, the flesh should be white with no brown stains.

----

detox ELIXIR

Push ½ a trimmed and coarsely chopped small beetroot (50g), 1 coarsely chopped small apple (130g), ½ a trimmed and coarsely chopped celery stalk (75g), ¼ cup firmly packed flat-leaf parsley leaves and ½ lemon (70g) through a juice extractor into a jug. Pour into serving glasses or bottles.

----

prep time 5 minutes
serves 1 (330ml)
nutritional count per serving protein (2.4g), carbohydrate (17g), total fat (0.3g), fibre (6g).

cook's notes

When pineapple is in season and at its best, it's a good idea to buy in bulk and freeze it. To freeze, peel and chop pineapple and freeze in sealed plastic bags for up to 3 months. If using frozen pineapple, you may need to use a little more as freezing can dilute the flavour.

"What you feed yourself today can improve all of your tomorrows."

METABOLISM-BOOSTER ELIXIR

DETOX ELIXIR

glow ELIXIR

Blend ½ cup (180g) coarsely chopped spinach, ⅔ cup (180ml) filtered water or coconut water, ½ a coarsely chopped lebanese cucumber (65g), ½ a coarsely chopped small apple (65g), ½ a coarsely chopped small carrot (35g), 6 fresh mint leaves and ¼ small avocado (50g) in a high-speed blender until smooth. Pour into serving glasses or bottles.

prep time 5 minutes
serves 2 (about 80ml each)
nutritional count per serving protein (3.3g), carbohydrate (5.9g), total fat (4.2g), fibre (4.1g).

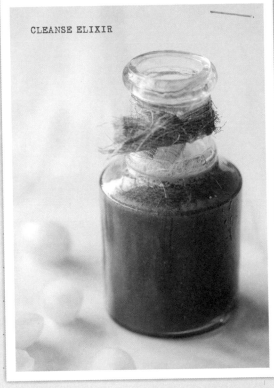

CLEANSE ELIXIR

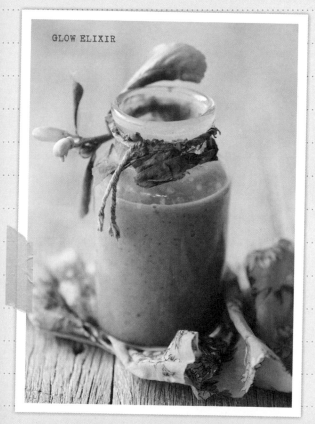

GLOW ELIXIR

cleanse ELIXIR

Push 1 trimmed and chopped medium kale leaf (40g), ½ a coarsely chopped lebanese cucumber (65g), ½ cup (75g) seedless green grapes and ¼ of a lime through a juice extractor into jug. Pour into serving glasses or bottles.

prep time 5 minutes
serves 2 (about 80ml each)
nutritional count per serving protein (0.8g), carbohydrate (6.8g), total fat (0.1g), fibre (1.2g).

balance ELIXIR

Blend 1 cup (250ml) almond or macadamia mylk with 2 seeded and chopped fresh dates, 1 teaspoon maca powder and ½ teaspoon vanilla bean paste, on high speed, until smooth. Pour into serving glasses or bottles.

----

prep time 5 minutes
serves 2 (about 125ml each)
nutritional count per serving protein (3.2g), carbohydrate (9.8g), total fat (9.2g), fibre (2.4g).

cook's notes

The word 'mylk' is used here to mean any non-dairy milk. See page 242 for our own macadamia mylk recipe.

Maca powder is the dried and ground root of the maca plant. It is high in antioxidants and vitamins. Available from health food stores.

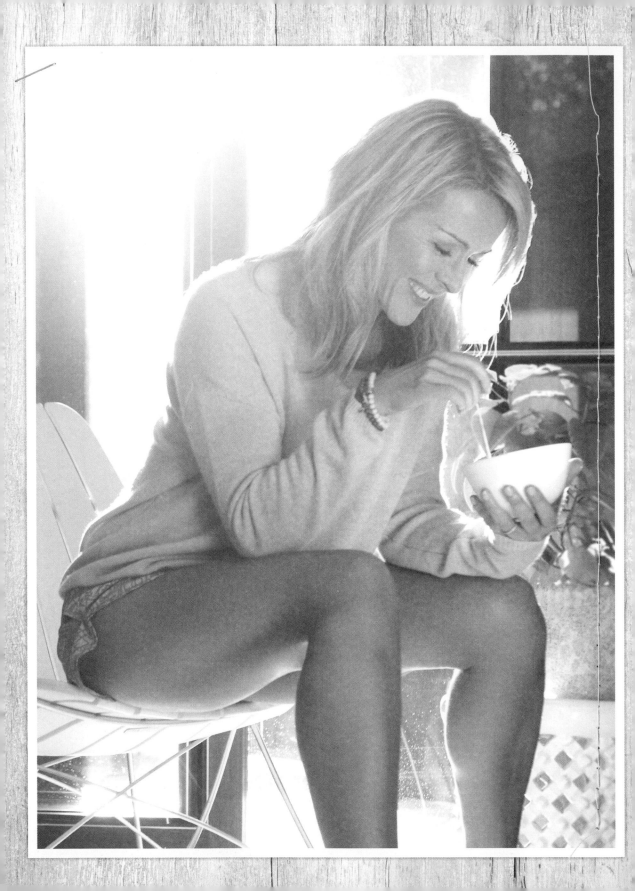

BREAKFAST

Breakfast is undoubtedly the most important meal of the day. From a quick, healthy energy bar or nutritious smoothie, to a leisurely brunch, this meal jump-starts our metabolism, gives us energy, makes us alert and puts us in a good mood for the rest of the day.

Now we all know how easy it is to skip breakfast, so the key is to find something that works for you and your morning routine.

In this section, you'll find a wide variety of my favourite breakfast options, some of which can be prepared ahead of time to grab and go, and others that are perfect to enjoy with family and friends when you have a little more time.

fruit salad with passionfruit yoghurt

1 medium kiwifruit (170g),
halved, sliced thinly

2 medium fresh figs (120g), quartered

1 pink grapefruit (350g), segmented

1 medium yellow nectarine (170g),
seeded, cut into thin wedges

¼ small rockmelon (300g),
peeled, seeded, chopped coarsely

65g (2 ounces) strawberries,
trimmed, halved

65g (2 ounces) raspberries

65g (2 ounces) blueberries

2 tablespoons lime juice

2 tablespoons loosely packed
fresh mint leaves

PASSIONFRUIT YOGHURT

⅔ cup (190g) unsweetened
greek yoghurt

⅓ cup (80ml) passionfruit pulp

2 teaspoons finely grated lime rind

1 Combine fruit and juice in a medium
bowl; toss gently to combine. Serve fruit
salad sprinkled with mint and
passionfruit yoghurt.

2 To make passionfruit yoghurt, combine
the ingredients in a small bowl and spoon
onto fruit salad.

prep time 15 minutes **serves** 2
nutritional count per serving (with yoghurt,
without syrup) protein (11.8g), carbohydrate
(51.5g), total fat (6.8g), fibre (18.5g).

cook's notes

You can use any combination of
fruit you like; choose whatever
is in season as it will be at its
best and most nutritious.

···········

You could serve this fruit salad
with a green tea, lemon grass
and ginger syrup. To make,
combine ½ cup (125ml) filtered
water, 2 tablespoons raw honey,
a thinly sliced 10cm (4-inch)
stick fresh lemon grass, a thinly
sliced 2.5cm (1-inch) piece fresh
ginger and 1 green tea bag in a
small saucepan; bring to the
boil. Boil uncovered for about
5 minutes or until syrup is
thickened slightly. Strain syrup
into a small jug; cool. Gently
toss the fruit salad with the cold
syrup just before serving.

···········

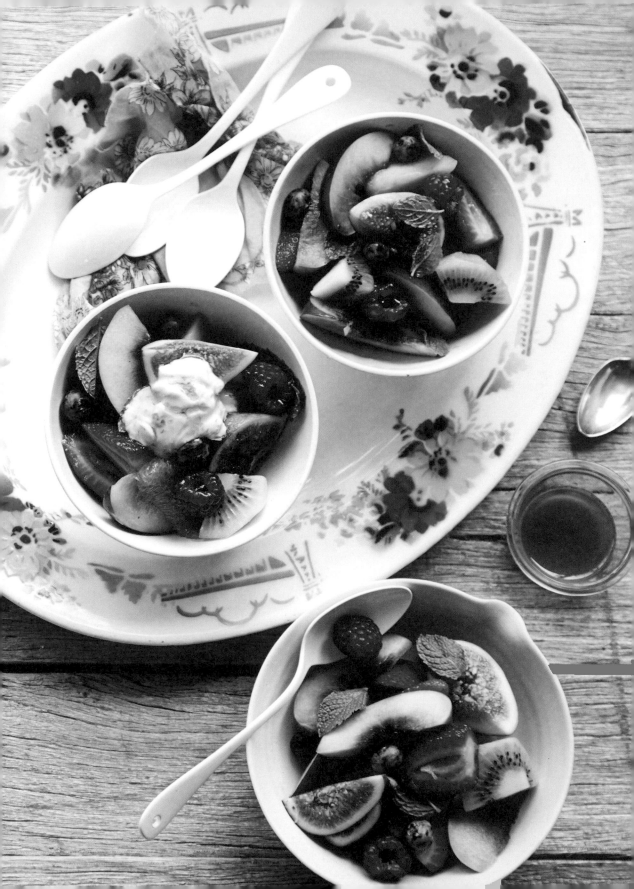

> "BREAKFAST IS THE MOST IMPORTANT MEAL OF THE DAY AND IT'S WORTH GETTING UP 15 MINUTES EARLIER TO MAKE SOMETHING NOURISHING AND DELICIOUS TO SAVOUR AT HOME OR TAKE TO WORK."

FIG, MACADAMIA AND HONEY PARFAIT

BLUEBERRY, PASSIONFRUIT & COCONUT PARFAIT

BERRIES AND YOGHURT PARFAIT

OVERNIGHT OATS PARFAIT WITH BERRIES AND YOGHURT

½ cup (45g) rolled oats

½ cup (40g) white quinoa flakes

1 tablespoon each pepitas (pumpkin seeds) and sunflower seed kernels

1 tablespoon black chia seeds

1½ teaspoons ground cinnamon

½ teaspoon ground nutmeg

1 cup (250ml) filtered water or macadamia mylk

1 tablespoon pure maple syrup

½ teaspoon vanilla bean paste or extract

½ cup (65g) halved strawberries

½ cup (65g) raspberries

½ cup (75g) blueberries

1 cup (280g) unsweetened greek yoghurt

1 Combine oats, quinoa, seeds, spices, water or mylk, maple syrup and vanilla in a medium bowl; cover; refrigerate overnight.

2 Smash half the berries with a fork. Layer oat mixture, yoghurt and smashed berries in 2 x 1¾ cup (430ml) serving glasses. Top with remaining whole berries.

prep time 15 minutes (+ refrigeration)
serves 2
nutritional count per serving
(with water) protein (19.7g), carbohydrate (63.2g), total fat (22g), fibre (8.2g).
(with macadamia mylk) protein (21.7g), carbohydrate (64.4g), total fat (42.1g), fibre (9.8g).

VARIATIONS

pear and chocolate

Replace berries with 1 thinly sliced or coarsely grated medium pear. Layer oat mixture and yoghurt with pear and 2 tablespoons cacao nibs.

blueberry, passionfruit & coconut

Instead of raspberries and strawberries, increase blueberries to 125g (4 ounces). Stir 2 teaspoons melted and cooled coconut oil into yoghurt. Layer oat mixture and yoghurt with blueberries and the pulp from 2 passionfruit. Sprinkle parfaits with 2 tablespoons toasted flaked coconut.

fig, macadamia and honey

Replace berries with 2 medium fresh figs, quartered. Layer oat mixture and yoghurt with figs, 2 teaspoons honey and 2 tablespoons coarsely chopped roasted macadamia nuts.

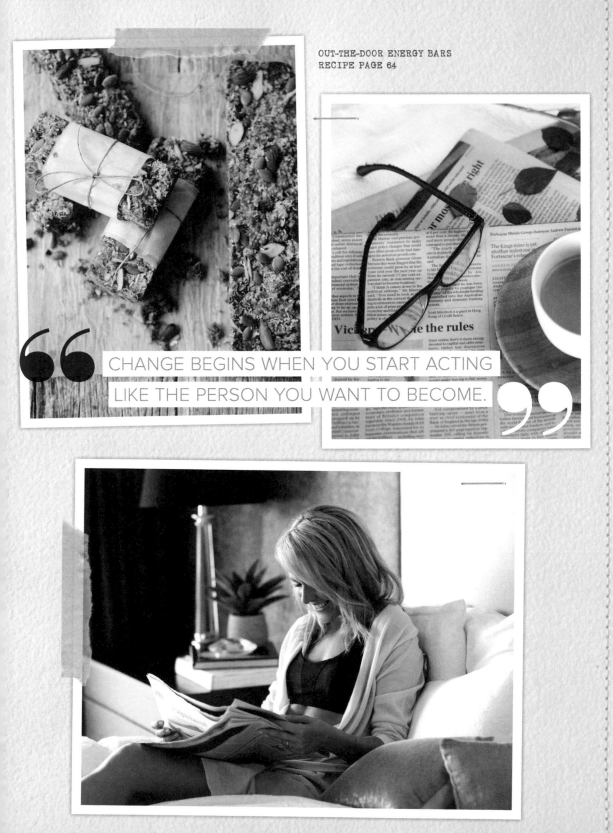

OUT-THE-DOOR ENERGY BARS
RECIPE PAGE 64

"CHANGE BEGINS WHEN YOU START ACTING LIKE THE PERSON YOU WANT TO BECOME."

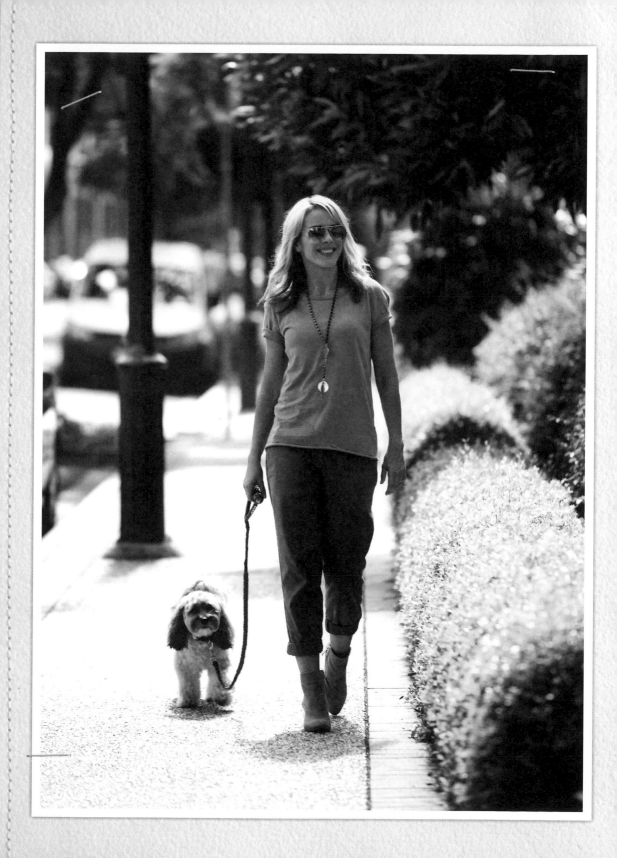

granola with cinnamon pears and coconut yoghurt

¾ cup (60g) quinoa flakes

¾ cup (70g) rolled oats

½ cup (75g) sunflower seed kernels

½ cup (100g) pepitas (pumpkin seeds)

½ cup (80g) almond kernels

½ cup (70g) hazelnuts

½ cup (25g) flaked coconut

½ teaspoon ground cinnamon

¼ cup (60ml) pure maple syrup

1 tablespoon cold-pressed extra-virgin coconut oil

⅓ cup (45g) dried goji berries

CINNAMON PEARS

1 medium pear (230g), quartered, cored

1 cinnamon stick

1 tablespoon raw honey

2 teaspoons lemon juice

¾ cup (180ml) filtered water

COCONUT YOGHURT

1 fresh young drinking coconut or ⅔ cup (400ml) canned coconut cream

1 vanilla bean, scraped

1 sachet (1 teaspoon) kefir powder or 1 teaspoon dairy-free high-strength probiotic powder (or 1 capsule)

1 To make coconut yoghurt, pour the water from the drinking coconut into a blender (you should have about 1¼ cups).

2 Using a spoon or ice-cream scoop, scoop out flesh from coconut; add to blender. Blend coconut mixture about 5 minutes or until smooth and creamy. Transfer to a sterilised jar; stir in vanilla and kefir powder or probiotic powder (or empty the contents of the capsule). Seal jar; stand mixture at room temperature 24 hours. Stir yoghurt; refrigerate until ready to use.

3 Preheat oven to 200°C/400°F. Combine quinoa, oats, seeds, nuts, coconut and spice in a medium bowl. Add combined maple syrup and oil; mix well. Spread mixture onto baking-paper-lined oven tray. Bake about 15 minutes or until browned lightly and crisp. Remove from oven; stir in berries. Cool granola on tray, stirring occasionally.

4 To make cinnamon pears, combine pear, cinnamon, honey, juice and water in a small saucepan; bring to the boil. Reduce heat; simmer, covered, 5 minutes or until pear is almost tender. Uncover; simmer 5 minutes or until pear is tender and syrup thickens slightly.

5 Serve ½ cup granola per person with pears, syrup and coconut yoghurt. Store remaining granola in an airtight container, in a cool dark place, for up to 2 weeks.

prep + cook time 45 minutes (+ cooling)
serves 2 (granola makes 4 cups; yoghurt makes about 2 cups)
nutritional count per serving protein (18.3g), carbohydrate (74g), total fat (49.7g), fibre (8.8g).

You will need to start making this recipe at least 24 hours ahead.

GRANOLA

cook's notes

Homemade coconut yoghurt is thinner than store-bought, but will thicken after 24 hours of refrigeration. If you want a thicker yoghurt, carefully scoop off the top thicker layer and discard water on the bottom. Yoghurt will keep in the fridge for up to 4 days.

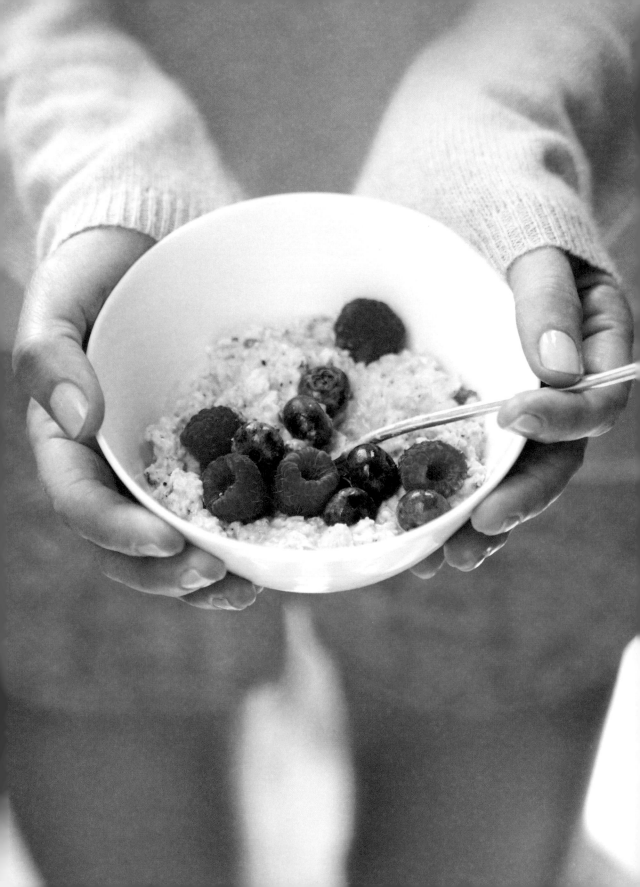

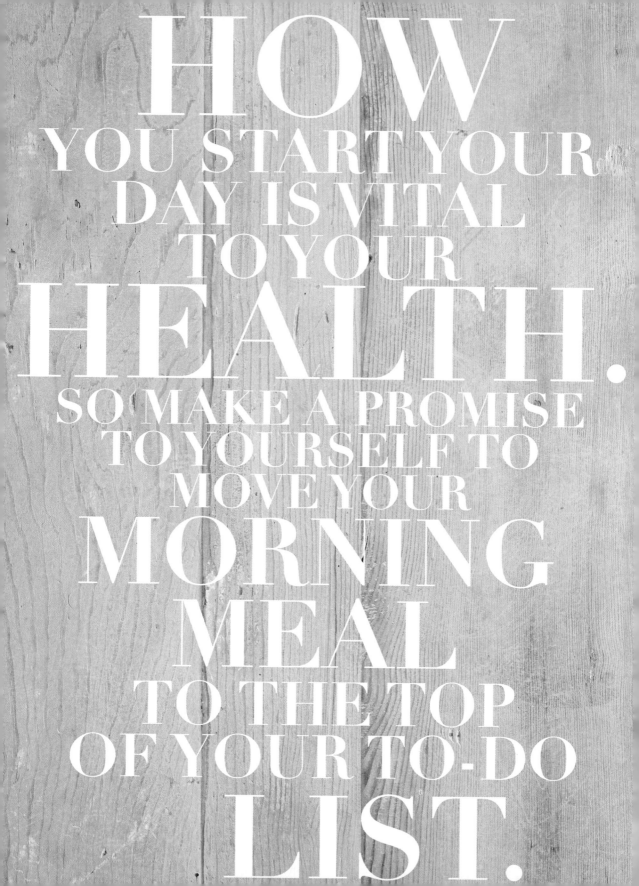

HOW YOU START YOUR DAY IS VITAL TO YOUR HEALTH. SO MAKE A PROMISE TO YOURSELF TO MOVE YOUR MORNING MEAL TO THE TOP OF YOUR TO-DO LIST.

out-the-door energy bars

1 cup (200g) pepitas (pumpkin seeds)

1 cup (160g) almond kernels

1 cup (90g) rolled oats

¾ cup (65g) natural wholegrain brown rice protein powder

½ cup (40g) desiccated coconut

½ cup (125g) cold-pressed extra-virgin coconut oil

½ cup (180g) raw honey

2 organic free-range eggs

⅓ cup (95g) natural peanut butter

⅓ cup (50g) cacao nibs

1 tablespoon bee pollen

2 teaspoons ground cinnamon

⅓ cup (40g) dried goji berries

1 tablespoon extra pepitas, rolled oats, desiccated coconut

1 Preheat oven to 160°C/325°F. Grease a shallow 22cm (9-inch) square cake pan; line base and sides with baking paper, extending paper 5cm (2 inches) over long sides.

2 Process pepitas, nuts, oats, protein powder, coconut, coconut oil, honey, eggs, peanut butter, cacao nibs, bee pollen and cinnamon until combined but still coarse. Stir in berries. Press mixture firmly into pan; sprinkle with extra pepitas, oats, coconut and nuts; press down firmly.

3 Bake about 30 minutes or until browned lightly (you may need to cover the pan with some aluminium foil if slice is becoming too brown). Cool in pan before cutting into bars.

prep + cook time 50 minutes (+ cooling)
makes 10 slices
nutritional count per serving protein (19.4g), carbohydrate (32.5g), total fat (40.7g), fibre (1.6g).

cook's notes

These bars are the perfect nutrient-dense, on-the-go breakfast for those mornings when you are running late. Bars will keep in an airtight container for up to 1 week; or freeze for up to 3 months. Take them out as you need them; they defrost at room temperature in minutes.

"LOADED WITH NUTRIENTS, THESE BARS HAVE NUTS FOR PROTEIN, CACAO NIBS FOR ENERGY AND CHEWY GOJI BERRIES FOR ANTIOXIDANTS."

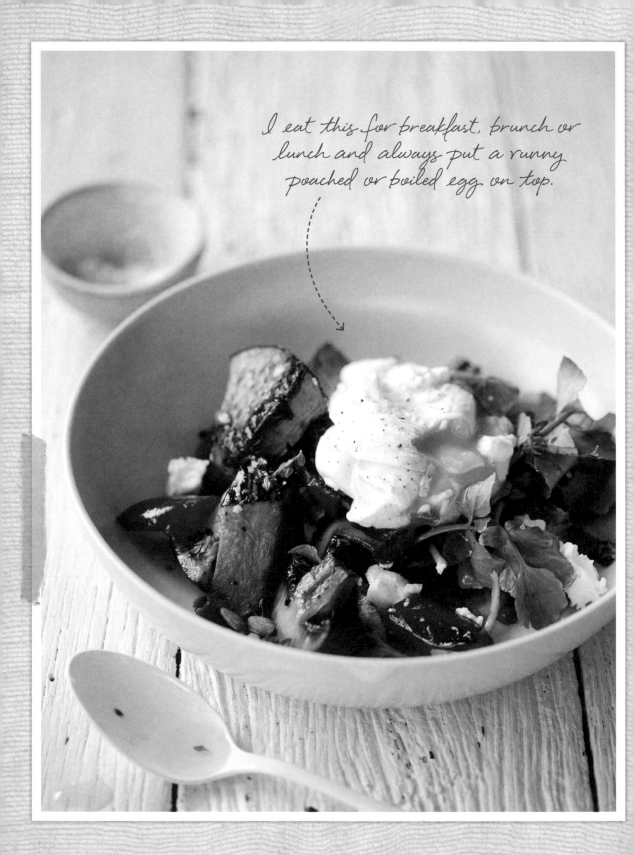

I eat this for breakfast, brunch or lunch and always put a runny poached or boiled egg on top.

nourishing
breakfast
salad

300g (9½-ounce) piece pumpkin, unpeeled, cut into 1cm (½-inch) thick slices

100g (3 ounces) swiss brown mushrooms, halved

1 large zucchini (180g), cut diagonally into 1cm (½-inch) thick slices

1 small red capsicum (bell pepper) (150g), sliced thickly

3 cups trimmed watercress leaves

1 tablespoon toasted pepitas (pumpkin seeds)

LEMON AND THYME DRESSING

1 tablespoon cold-pressed extra-virgin coconut oil

1½ tablespoons lemon juice

2 teaspoons fresh thyme leaves

2 teaspoons pure maple syrup

1 Preheat oven to 220°C/425°F.
2 To make lemon and thyme dressing, combine the ingredients in a screw-top jar and season to taste. Shake well.
3 Combine vegetables and 1 tablespoon dressing in a large baking-paper-lined baking dish. Bake about 25 minutes or until vegetables are browned lightly and tender.
4 Combine vegetables and watercress in large bowl. Transfer to serving plates; sprinkle with pepitas. Drizzle with remaining dressing.

prep + cook time 35 minutes
serves 2
nutritional count per serving (without egg or cheese) protein (14.3g), carbohydrate (28.5g), total fat (13.8g), fibre (12.2g)
(with egg and cheese) protein (24.3g), carbohydrate (29.3g), total fat (23.2g), fibre (12.2g).

cook's notes

The best poached egg: bring a saucepan of water to the boil then reduce to a simmer. Crack an egg into a cup and slide into the water in the centre of the pan. Cook 5 minutes or until the eggs are cooked to your liking, and remove with a slotted spoon.

You can use any combination of vegetables you like; just try to use the same weight.

You can roast the vegetables the night before and store in an airtight container in the fridge. Reheat them just before serving, or use them cold if you prefer. For an added protein hit, you can sprinkle salad with a little goat's cheese.

Don't deprive yourself of the things you love; and never, ever forget that food is meant to be nourishing but should also be celebrated and enjoyed.

smashed eggs with spinach on toast

1 teaspoon cold-pressed
extra virgin coconut oil

1 green onion (scallions), sliced thinly

80g (2½ ounces) baby spinach leaves

2 teaspoons each
finely chopped fresh dill and mint

4 organic free-range eggs

4 slices (300g)
MNB seed and nut bread

1 medium lemon (140g),
cut into wedges

Micro herbs, to garnish

1 Heat oil in a medium frying pan; cook onion, stirring, until onion softens. Add spinach; stir until wilted. Remove from heat; stir in herbs, season to taste. Transfer to small bowl; cover to keep warm.

2 Cover eggs with cold water in a small saucepan; bring to the boil. Boil, uncovered, about 3 minutes or until soft boiled. When eggs are cool enough to handle, peel eggs.

3 Meanwhile, toast bread. Serve toast topped with spinach mixture and chopped eggs. Serve with lemon wedges and micro herbs.

prep + cook time 25 minutes
serves 2
nutritional count per serving protein (35.4g), carbohydrate (20.9g), total fat (50.6g), fibre (4g).

cook's notes

You'll find the recipe for our homemade MNB seed and nut bread on page 240. Alternatively, you can use a spelt-flour, dark rye or wholegrain sourdough bread as a good substitute.

Eggs are the perfect breakfast
food as they are protein-
packed to keep you
fuller for longer.

"EXPECT THE MOST
WONDERFUL
THINGS
TO HAPPEN,
NOT IN THE
FUTURE,
BUT
RIGHT
NOW."

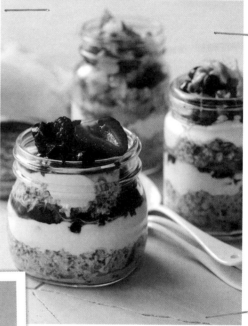

OVERNIGHT OATS PARFAIT
WITH BERRIES AND
YOGHURT RECIPE PAGE 57

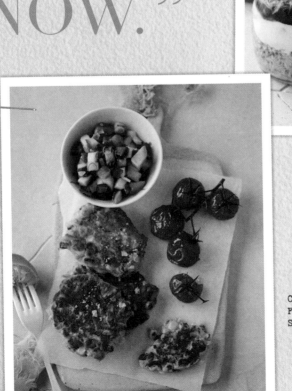

CORN AND CAPSICUM
FRITTERS WITH AVOCADO
SALSA RECIPE PAGE 78

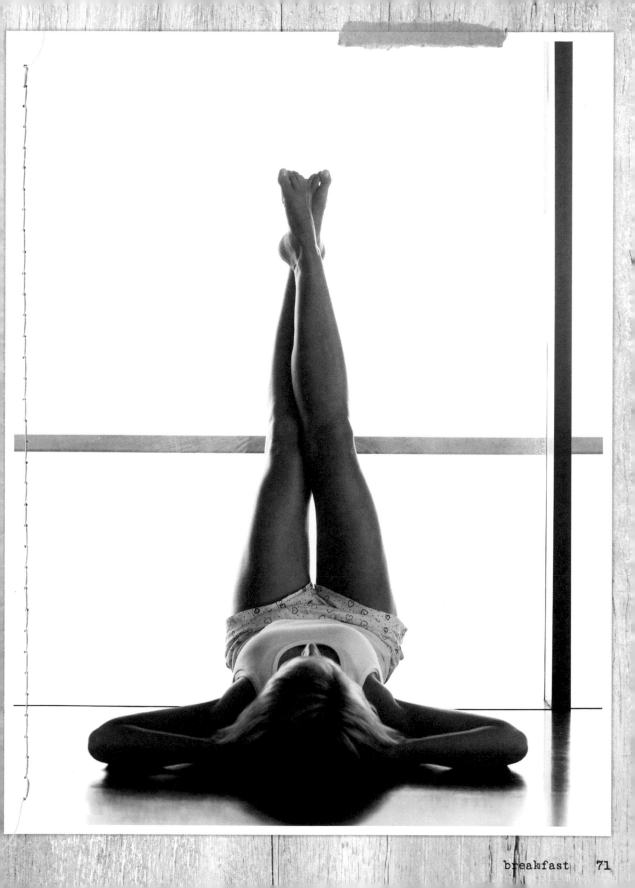

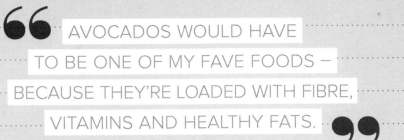

ROASTED BALSAMIC TOMATO AND AVOCADO ON TOAST

250g (8 ounces) cherry truss tomatoes

1 tablespoon balsamic vinegar

4 slices MNB seed and nut bread
2cm (¾-inch) thick (300g)

125g (2 ounces) rocket (arugula), trimmed

1 medium avocado (250g), sliced thinly

2 tablespoons coarsely chopped
roasted walnuts

50g (1½ ounces) soft goat's cheese

1 Preheat oven to 220°C/425°F.

2 Combine tomatoes and vinegar in a large
baking-paper-lined baking dish; season to
taste. Bake about 10 minutes or until tomatoes
are browned lightly and beginning to soften.

3 Meanwhile, toast bread. Serve toast topped
with rocket, avocado and tomato; sprinkle
with nuts and cheese, drizzle with any pan
juices from tomatoes.

prep + cook time 30 minutes
serves 2
nutritional count per serving protein (31.2g),
carbohydrate (23.4g), total fat (69.9g), fibre (10g).

cook's notes

We all know that avocados and
tomatoes are delicious – cooked
or raw – but did you know they
are two of our most versatile
superfoods! Loaded with
vitamins, minerals and
antioxidants, they are nature's
own beauty treatments.
While avocado can be used
topically on the skin to soften
and moisturise, or even help
repair damaged hair, including
lycopene-rich tomatoes in your
diet has been shown to protect
the skin from free radicals and
UV damage.

cook's notes

We used homemade MNB seed and nut bread (see page 240 for this recipe) but you can use a spelt flour, dark rye or wholegrain sourdough bread.

I love to spread my toast with a little Vegemite (underneath the avocado) to stock up on my B-group vitamins and help keep my mid-morning sugar cravings at bay.

----

omelettes with 3 fillings

See following pages for recipes

cook's notes

By using the basic omelette recipe on page 76, you can try these fillings and then develop your own combinations from your favourite foods and flavours.

MIXED MUSHROOM
AND HERB OMELETTE

ROASTED KUMARA, KALE
AND GOAT'S CHEESE
OMELETTE

cook's notes

The roasted kumara filling is
a great way to use left-over
vegetables from the night
before. Just keep to the
quantities in the recipe and
share your faves with me
@ljclarkson.

SALMON, SPINACH
AND PRESERVED
LEMON OMELETTE

omelettes with 3 fillings

basic omelette

1 teaspoon cold-pressed
extra virgin coconut oil
- -
4 organic free-range eggs
- -
1 tablespoon filtered water
- -

1 Prepare desired filling.
2 Heat half the oil in a small frying pan
(top measurement about 20cm/8 inches).
Whisk eggs and the water in a medium
jug until frothy. Pour half the egg mixture
into pan; cook omelette over medium
heat until omelette is just beginning to
set around the edges. Top with desired
filling; continue cooking until omelette is
just set. Carefully slide omelette onto
plate, cover to keep warm.
3 Repeat with remaining oil, egg
mixture and desired filling to make
another omelette.
- -
prep + cook time 25 minutes
serves 2

roasted kumara, kale and goat's cheese omelette

Before making the omelettes, preheat
oven to 200°C/400°F. Chop ½ medium
kumara (orange sweet potato) into 1.5cm
(¾-inch) pieces. Place on baking-paper-
lined oven tray; drizzle with ½ teaspoon
coconut oil. Roast about 15 minutes or
until browned lightly and tender. Heat
½ teaspoon of oil in the omelette frying
pan; cook 2 trimmed and chopped kale
leaves, 30 seconds or until just tender,
remove from pan. Wipe pan clean, make
omelettes (see step 2, left); top with
kumara and kale, sprinkle with 60g
(2 ounces) soft goat's cheese. Continue
cooking until omelette is set.
- -
**roasted kumara, kale and goat's cheese
nutritional count per serving** protein
(20.4g), carbohydrate (13.8g), total fat
(21.3g), fibre (2.4g).

salmon, spinach and preserved lemon omelette

Place 1 x 150g (4½-ounce) boneless salmon fillet, with skin on, in a baking-paper-lined bamboo steamer; add 5cm (2-inch) strip preserved lemon rind. Set the steamer over a small saucepan of boiling water; steam salmon, covered, about 10 minutes or until cooked as desired. Remove from heat. Discard skin; flake salmon. Make omelettes (see step 2, opposite); sprinkle with 1 cup (40g) loosely packed baby spinach leaves, flaked salmon, 1 tablespoon rinsed and drained baby capers and 1 tablespoon finely shredded preserved lemon rind. Continue cooking until omelette is set. Serve sprinkled with a pinch of cayenne pepper and lemon wedges, if you like.

- -

salmon, spinach and preserved lemon nutritional count per serving protein (34.8g), carbohydrate (2.6g), total fat (22.2g), fibre (0.1g).

mixed mushroom and herb omelette

Before making the omelettes, heat 2 teaspoons coconut oil in the frying pan and cook 300g (9½ ounces) coarsely chopped mixed mushrooms (we used swiss brown, flat, oyster and enoki mushrooms) and 1 crushed garlic clove, stirring, until golden and tender. Wipe the pan clean and make omelettes (see step 2, opposite); sprinkle with 1 tablespoon finely chopped fresh herbs (we used parsley and chives) and top with mushroom mixture. Continue cooking until omelette is set. Serve sprinkled with micro/baby herbs of your choice and lemon wedges.

- -

mixed mushroom and herb nutritional count per serving
protein (18.4g), carbohydrate (4.2g), total fat (17.8g), fibre (4.3g).

corn and capsicum fritters with avocado salsa

250g (8 ounces) cherry truss tomatoes

¼ cup (35g) brown rice flour

¼ cup (35g) chick pea (garbanzo/besan) flour

1 teaspoon baking powder

½ teaspoon each
ground cumin and ground coriander

pinch ground cayenne pepper

1 organic free-range egg

⅓ cup (80ml) filtered water

2 cups (280g) fresh corn kernels

1 large red capsicum (bell pepper),
chopped finely

1 green onion (scallion), chopped finely

2 teaspoons cold-pressed
extra virgin coconut oil

AVOCADO AND CUCUMBER SALSA

1 medium avocado (250g),
cut into 1cm (½-inch) pieces

1 lebanese cucumber (130g),
cut into 1cm (½-inch) pieces

½ small red capsicum (bell pepper),
chopped finely

⅓ cup loosely packed
fresh coriander (cilantro) leaves

1 tablespoon lime juice

1 green onion (scallion), chopped finely

1 Preheat oven to 200°C/400°F.

2 Cut tomatoes into 2 bundles. Place tomatoes on oven tray; season. Bake about 10 minutes or until skins burst.

3 Meanwhile, sift flours, baking powder and spices into a medium bowl; gradually whisk in combined egg and water until batter is smooth. Stir in corn, capsicum and onion; season to taste.

4 Heat half the oil in a large frying pan; pour ¼ cup batter for each fritter into pan, using spatula, spread into round shape. (You can cook 3-4 fritters at a time). Cook fritters about 2 minutes each side or until browned and cooked through. Remove from pan; cover to keep warm. Repeat with remaining oil and batter to make a total of 6 fritters.

5 Meanwhile, to make avocado and cucumber salsa, combine ingredients in a small bowl. Season to taste.

6 Serve fritters with salsa and tomatoes. Sprinkle with extra fresh coriander leaves, if you like.

prep + cook time 40 minutes
serves 2
nutritional count per serving protein (18.5g), carbohydrate (47g), total fat (32.3g), fibre (17.6g).

These fritters make a delicious snack, they're amazing hot or cold and are great for fighting afternoon hunger pains.

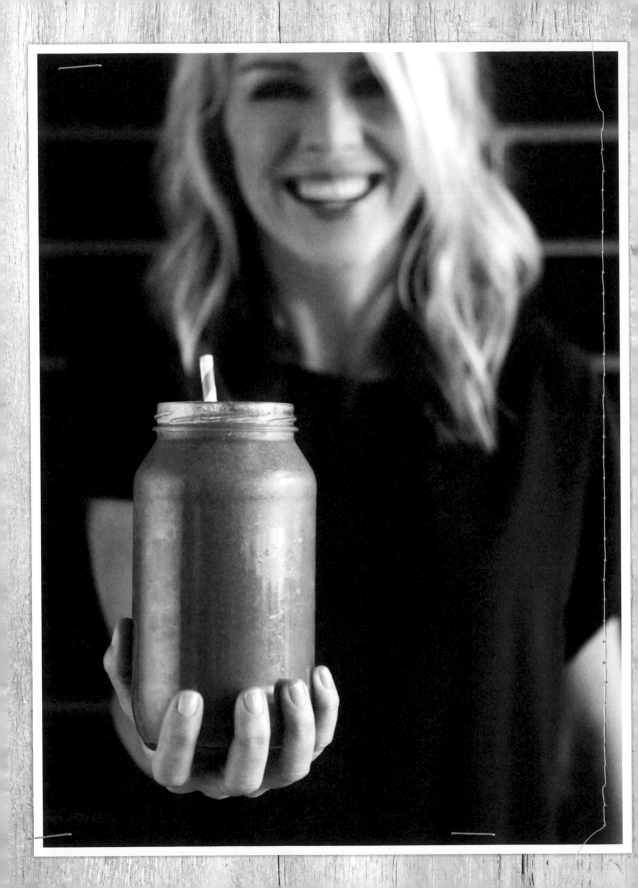

SMOOTHIES

Smoothies are a great way to get more nutrition into our diets. With many people not eating enough fruit and vegetables, smoothies are also quick and easy to prepare and packed with nutrients. They can be customised for maximum benefits and are absolutely delicious.

I LOVE a good smoothie - what I enjoy most about them is that the combinations are limited only by your imagination, and you can address unlimited health concerns with the ingredients you choose to include. From boosting your immunity, to improving your skin, getting an extra boost of energy or your daily recommended dose of antioxidants there is a smoothie just for YOU!

The smoothie recipes in this book are some of my favourites and each one serves its own purpose. Pick the ones that work for you and enjoy them when and wherever you can.

green smoothies

Green smoothies are a delicious way to bump up your daily intake of green goodness - and the more leafy greens you can get into your smoothie the better! But let me warn you, they are an acquired taste so my suggestion is you start with a little more fruit and over time, start to reduce it to eventually reduce your overall sugar intake.

To help you with this exercise I have included 4 variations for my green smoothies - from Mild (with more fruit) to Hardcore (as the name insinuates - no fruit at all). I suggest if you are new to green smoothies, start with Mild and feel free to adjust the fruit content as you wish ... with the ultimate goal over time to enjoy and look forward to the strong hardcore versions that make an almost daily appearance on my desk at work.

So go ahead and give green smoothies a try - they are perfect for days when you have a lot planned; you can simply pour all of the things you know are good for you into a blender and enjoy its nutritional goodness all morning long.

green smoothie 1 (MILD)

In a high speed blender, blend 1½ cups loosely packed baby spinach leaves, 1 coarsely chopped small banana (130g), ½ peeled, cored and coarsely chopped medium ripe pear (115g), 1 peeled, seeded and coarsely chopped small orange (180g), ½ coarsely chopped lebanese cucumber (65g) and ½ cup (125ml) filtered water or coconut water until smooth. Serve in glass.

- -

prep time 5 minutes **serves** 1 (375ml)
nutritional count per serving (with water)
protein (5.6g), carbohydrate (43.1g), total fat (0.7g), fibre (8g); (with coconut water) protein (6.3g), carbohydrate (49.1g), total fat (0.8g), fibre (8g).

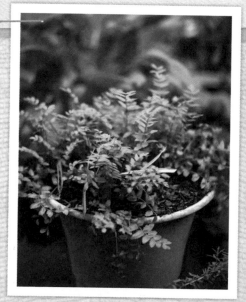

GREEN SMOOTHIE 1 (MILD)

green smoothies

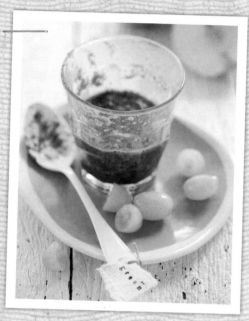

green smoothie 2 (MODERATE)

Wash and trim 2 medium kale leaves (80g), discarding stalks. Chop leaves coarsely. In a high speed blender, blend kale with 1 peeled, cored and coarsely chopped medium green-skinned apple (150g), 1 cup (175g) seedless green grapes, 8 fresh mint leaves and ½ cup (125ml) filtered water or coconut water until smooth. Serve in glass.

----

prep time 5 minutes **serves** 1 (375ml)
nutritional count per serving (with water) protein (3.5g), carbohydrate (41.3g), total fat (0.6g), fibre (7.3g); (with coconut water) protein (4.2g), carbohydrate (47.3g), total fat (0.8g), fibre (7.3g).

> " GREEN SMOOTHIES ARE A DAILY RITUAL FOR ME AND I'M SURE ONCE YOU FEEL THEIR BENEFITS, THEY'LL BE A NON-NEGOTIABLE PART OF YOUR DAY TOO. "

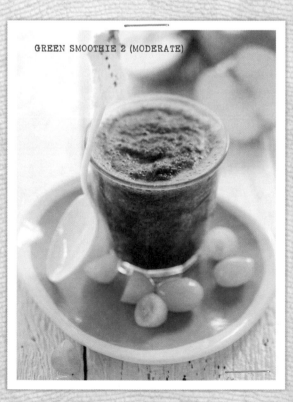

GREEN SMOOTHIE 2 (MODERATE)

cook's notes

Smoothies are best served chilled and will keep in a sealed glass jar for up to 2 days. Shake or stir before serving.

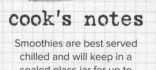

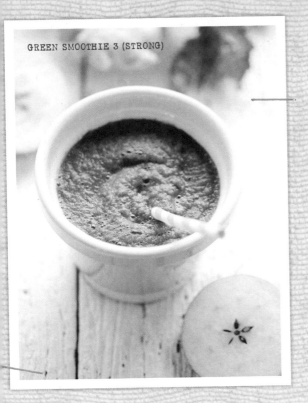

GREEN SMOOTHIE 3 (STRONG)

green smoothie 4 (HARDCORE)

Wash and trim 1 medium kale leaf (40g), discarding stalk; chop leaf coarsely. In a high speed blender, blend kale with ½ cup loosely packed baby spinach leaves, 1 coarsely chopped lebanese cucumber (130g), ⅓ cup loosely packed fresh flat-leaf parsley leaves, 2 tablespoons lemon juice, ½ teaspoon spirulina powder and ½ cup (125ml) filtered water or coconut water until smooth. Serve in glass.

prep time 5 minutes **serves** 1 (375ml)
nutritional count per serving (with water)
protein (3.3g), carbohydrate (5.3g), total fat
(0.4g), fibre (4.7g); (with coconut water)
protein (3.9g), carbohydrate (11.3g), total fat
(0.6g), fibre (4.7g).

green smoothie 3 (STRONG)

Wash, trim and coarsely chop 2 medium silver beet (swiss chard) leaves (130g), discarding white stalks. In a high speed blender, blend silver beet with 1 coarsely chopped celery stalk (150g), 1 peeled, cored and coarsely chopped, medium green-skinned apple (150g), 1 peeled, seeded and coarsely chopped medium orange (240g), grated 1cm (½-inch) piece fresh ginger (5g) and ½ cup (125ml) filtered water or coconut water until smooth. Serve in glass.

prep time 5 minutes **serves** 1 (375ml)
nutritional count per serving (with water) protein (4.4g), carbohydrate (27.1g), total fat (0.6g), fibre (9.4g); (with coconut water) protein (5g), carbohydrate (33.1g), total fat (0.7g), fibre (9.4g)

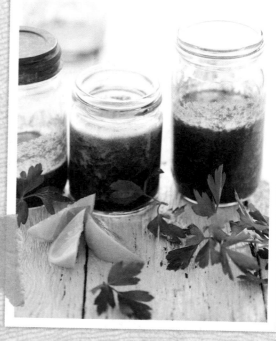

GREEN SMOOTHIE 4 (HARDCORE)

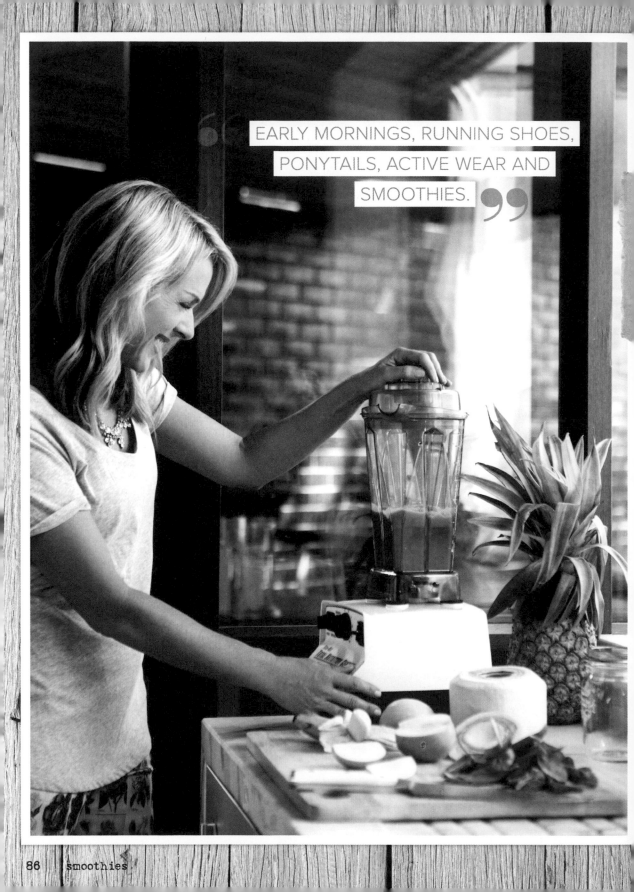

EARLY MORNINGS, RUNNING SHOES, PONYTAILS, ACTIVE WEAR AND SMOOTHIES.

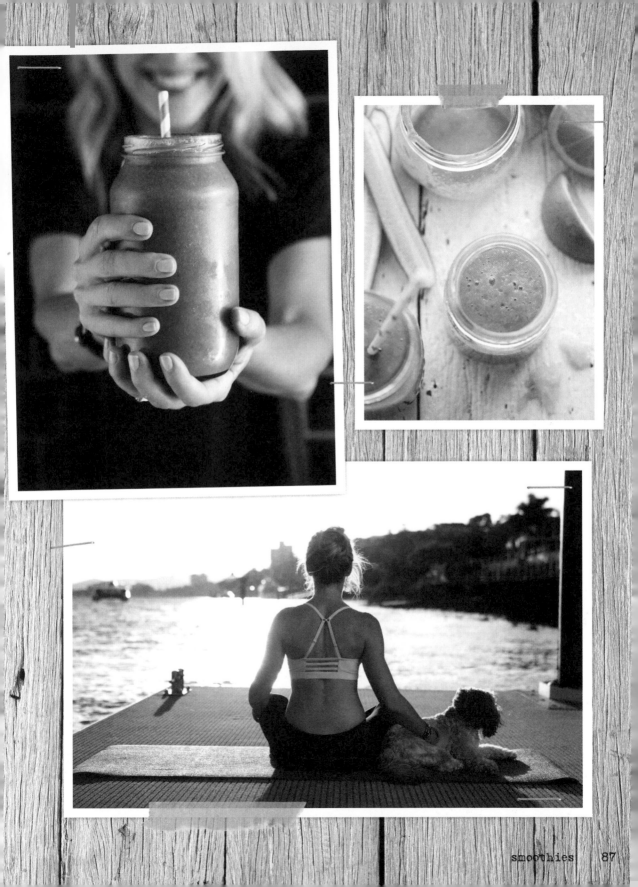

> "POUR ALL THE THINGS YOU KNOW ARE GOOD FOR YOU INTO A BLENDER AND ENJOY IT ALL MORNING LONG."

breakfast
smoothie

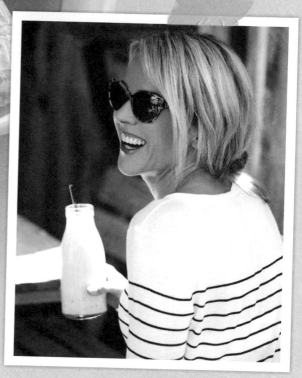

cook's notes

Chia seeds add thickness to a smoothie. They are also high in fibre, omega 3, antioxidants, protein, vitamin C, iron, calcium and potassium.

Blend 1 cup loosely packed baby spinach leaves, 1 coarsely chopped medium banana (200g), ½ coarsely chopped small mango (150g), 1 cup (250ml) macadamia mylk (see page 242), 1 tablespoon almond butter, 2 teaspoons white chia seeds, 2 teaspoons raw honey and 1 teaspoon maca powder until smooth. Serve in a glass sprinkled with 3 dried banana slices and ½ teaspoon each chia seeds and bee pollen.

prep time 5 minutes **serves** 1 (375ml)
nutritional count per serving protein (16.6g), carbohydrate (90.2g), total fat (67.7g), fibre (14.6g).

Spirulina is over 60 per cent protein and is packed with antioxidants.

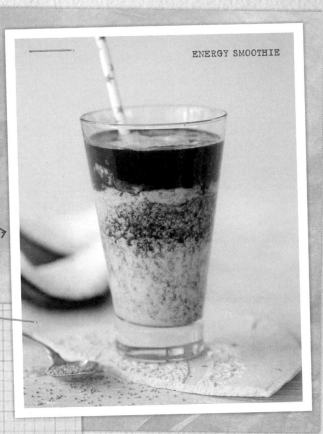

energy SMOOTHIE

Blend 1 coarsely chopped large banana (230g), 2 tablespoons macadamia nuts, 1 cup (250ml) pure coconut water, 2 teaspoons white chia seeds, 2 teaspoons pure maple syrup, 1 teaspoon ground cinnamon and 1 tablespoon melted and cooled cold-pressed, extra-virgin coconut oil until smooth. Pour into glass. Stand 2 minutes or until thickened. Combine 1 teaspoon spirulina powder with ⅓ cup (80ml) filtered water in a small jug. Carefully pour spirulina mixture on top of macadamia mixture.

prep time 5 minutes **serves** 1 (300ml)
nutritional count per serving protein (9.8g), carbohydrate (56.3g), total fat (39.1g), fibre (7.1g).

wonder woman SMOOTHIE

Trim, peel and coarsely chop ½ small beetroot (50g). Blend beetroot with 1 peeled, cored and coarsely chopped small apple (130g), ½ cup (60g) broccoli florets, ½ coarsely chopped small avocado (100g), ½ cup (75g) frozen mixed berries, ½ cup (125g) frozen chopped pineapple and ½ cup (125ml) macadamia mylk (see page 242) until smooth. Serve in glass topped with 1 teaspoon flaked coconut, 1 tablespoon blueberries and ½ teaspoon bee pollen.

prep time 10 minutes **serves** 1 (375ml)
nutritional count per serving protein (10.3g), carbohydrate (31.5g), total fat (38.1g), fibre (13.1g).

cook's notes

We used frozen pineapple but you can use fresh if you prefer; you will need about ¼ small pineapple.

Wear gloves when preparing the beetroot as it may stain your hands. Because of the hardy texture of the beetroot, this smoothie will take a little longer to blend until smooth.

WONDER WOMAN SMOOTHIE

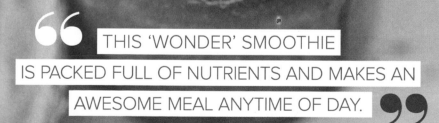

66 THIS 'WONDER' SMOOTHIE IS PACKED FULL OF NUTRIENTS AND MAKES AN AWESOME MEAL ANYTIME OF DAY. 99

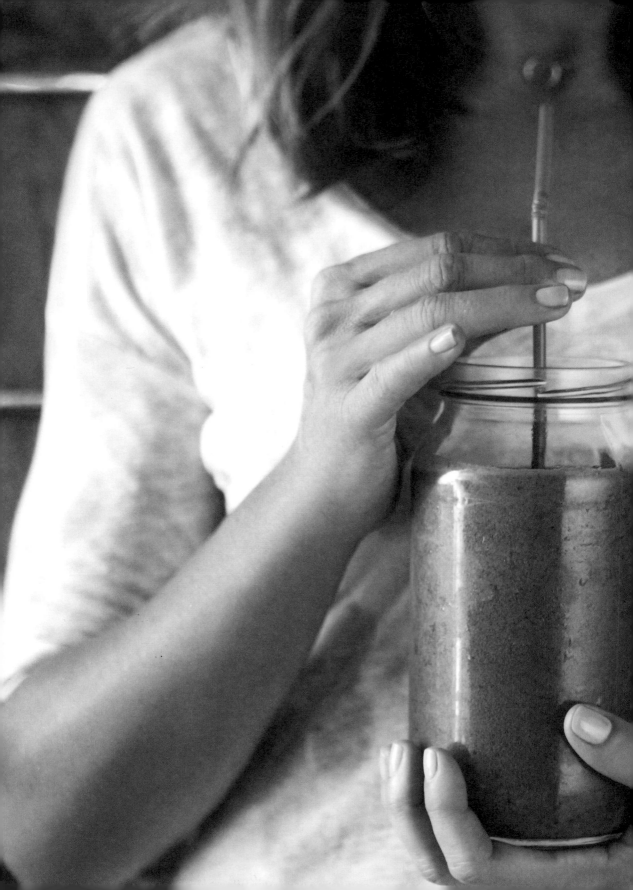

"EVERYONE DESERVES TO FEEL ENERGISED, VIBRANT AND FULL OF LIFE."

rescue
SMOOTHIE

Blend 1 cup (250g) frozen chopped pineapple, 1 cup (250ml) pure coconut water, ½ cup (140g) unsweetened greek yoghurt and 8 fresh mint leaves until smooth. Serve in glass topped with extra mint leaves, 2 teaspoons flaked coconut and 1 teaspoon passionfruit pulp.

----

prep time 5 minutes **serves** 1 (375ml)
nutritional count per serving protein (10.7g), carbohydrate (53.5g), total fat (11.9g), fibre (6.1g).

For a dairy-free option, replace the greek yoghurt with the same quantity of coconut yoghurt.

ultimate SMOOTHIE

Blend ½ cup (125ml) macadamia mylk (see page 242), ¾ cup (180ml) pure coconut water, ¼ cup young coconut flesh, 2 cups (300g) frozen mixed berries, 1 teaspoon vanilla bean paste or extract, 2 teaspoons protein powder, 2 teaspoons cacao powder and 1 teaspoon maca powder until smooth. Serve in glass topped with 1 teaspoon cacao nibs, 1 teaspoon toasted flaked coconut and 1 tablespoon extra berries.

----

prep time 5 minutes **serves** 1 (330ml)
nutritional count per serving protein (10g), carbohydrate (50.5g), total fat (25.5g), fibre (1.7g).

cook's notes

You will need 1 young drinking coconut for this recipe. We used both the pure coconut water and the soft jelly-like flesh (which we scooped out with a spoon). You can use extra coconut water instead of the macadamia mylk, if you prefer.

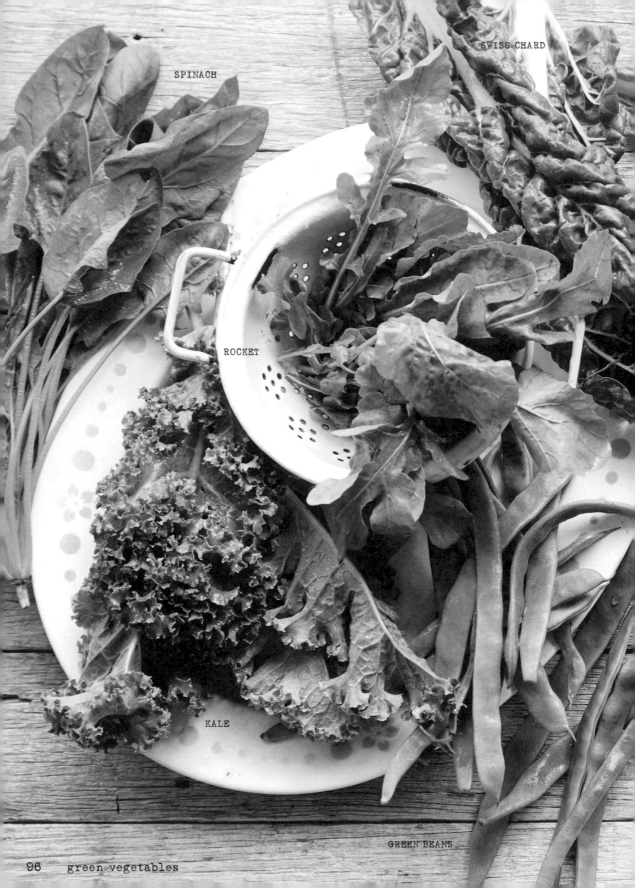

SPINACH

SWISS CHARD

ROCKET

KALE

GREEN BEANS

BEETROOT LEAVES

GREEN VEGETABLES
pack a powerful nutritional punch, especially when used as a key ingredient in smoothies. Here is a selection of my favourites.

TUSCAN KALE

SUNFLOWER SPROUTS

BROCCOLI

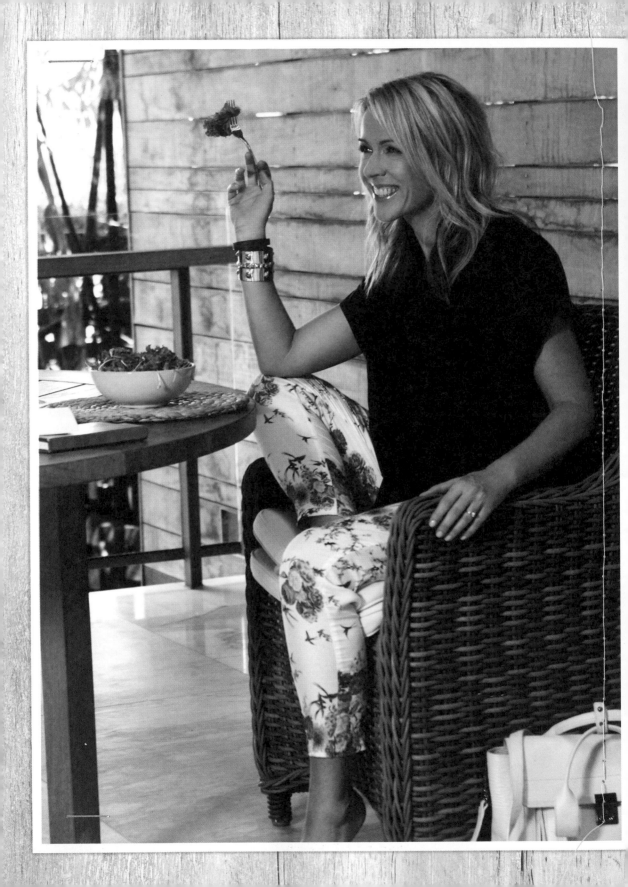

LUNCH

I make lunch for myself most days, preparing it in the morning or the night before and usually making a couple of lunches at a time.

On most days it will be a salad with protein, but sometimes I'll mix it up and have a soup with a smaller salad, nutrient-filled rice paper rolls or some homemade sushi.

I like to eat lunch where there is fresh air - near a window, on a verandah or sitting outside, but I often find myself at my desk through the week checking emails between mouthfuls 10 minutes before my next meeting!

No matter how busy I am, I always try to sit up straight, chew slowly, relax a little and enjoy my food.

Lunch is a great way to pause and re-fuel your body, so I hope the following recipes will inspire you to take the time to sit, re-charge and prepare yourself nutritionally for the second half of your day.

detox green soup

1 large green capsicum
(bell pepper) (350g)

2 cloves garlic, unpeeled

1 cup (125g) broccoli florets

1 teaspoon (20g) cold-pressed
extra-virgin coconut oil

2 lebanese cucumbers, chopped coarsely

1 cup (35g) baby spinach leaves

1 tablespoon lime juice

¼ cup (40g) almond kernels

¼ cup loosely packed
fresh coriander (cilantro) leaves

¼ cup loosely packed fresh mint leaves

AVOCADO AND LIME SALSA

½ small avocado (100g), chopped finely

1 green onion (scallion), chopped finely

2 teaspoons finely chopped
fresh coriander (cilantro)

2 teaspoons finely chopped fresh mint

1 tablespoon cold-pressed
extra-virgin coconut oil

1 tablespoon lime juice

1 Preheat oven to 200°C/400°F.
2 Combine capsicum, garlic and broccoli
with the oil in a small baking dish. Bake
about 10 minutes or until capsicum is just
tender. Cool.
3 Peel garlic. Blend garlic with the
remaining soup ingredients, in a high-speed
blender, until smooth. Strain mixture
through a fine sieve into large jug; cover;
refrigerate 3 hours or overnight.
4 To make the avocado and lime salsa,
combine all the ingredients in a small bowl;
season to taste.
5 Season soup to taste; pour into bowls.
Serve topped with avocado salsa.

prep + cook time 30 minutes (+ refrigeration)
serves 2
nutritional count per serving protein
(13.1g), carbohydrate (10.8g), total fat (28.2g),
fibre (10g).

Served hot or cold this soup is delightfully refreshing and cleansing.

dEtox soup

cook's notes

If you're taking this soup to work, pack the soup and salsa separately and assemble just before eating. Soup will keep in the fridge in an airtight container for up to 3 days. Avocado salsa is best made the day it is being served or it may go brown.

Soups are like smoothies – packed with nutrition and easy to digest.

KUMARA AND PEANUT BUTTER SOUP

1 tablespoon cold-pressed extra-virgin coconut oil

1 small brown onion (100g), finely chopped

2 cloves garlic, crushed

2.5cm (1-inch) piece fresh ginger (10g), grated

1 teaspoon ground cinnamon

1 small red capsicum (bell pepper) (150g), chopped coarsely

2 small kumara (orange sweet potato) (500g), chopped coarsely

1 medium tomato (150g), chopped coarsely

½ cup (140g) natural peanut butter

2½ cups (625ml) filtered water or coconut mylk (see page 242 for recipe)

50g (1½ ounces) green beans, trimmed, halved lengthways

½ fresh long red chilli, sliced thinly

⅓ cup loosely packed fresh coriander (cilantro) leaves

2 tablespoons roasted unsalted peanuts or cashews

1 lime, cut into wedges

1 Heat oil in a medium saucepan; cook onion, garlic and ginger, stirring, until onion softens. Add cinnamon; cook, stirring, 1 minute or until fragrant.
2 Add capsicum, kumara, tomato, peanut butter and the water; bring to the boil. Reduce heat; simmer, uncovered, 15 minutes or until kumara is tender. Cool soup 10 minutes.
3 Blend soup, in batches, until smooth.
4 Season soup to taste; ladle into serving bowls. Serve topped with beans, chilli, coriander, nuts and lime wedges.

prep + cook time 35 minutes
serves 2
nutritional count per serving (with water) protein (29.2g), carbohydrate (46.8g), total fat (50.8g), fibre (8.3g); (with coconut mylk) protein (30.7g), carbohydrate (67.7g), total fat (54.3g), fibre (8.6g).

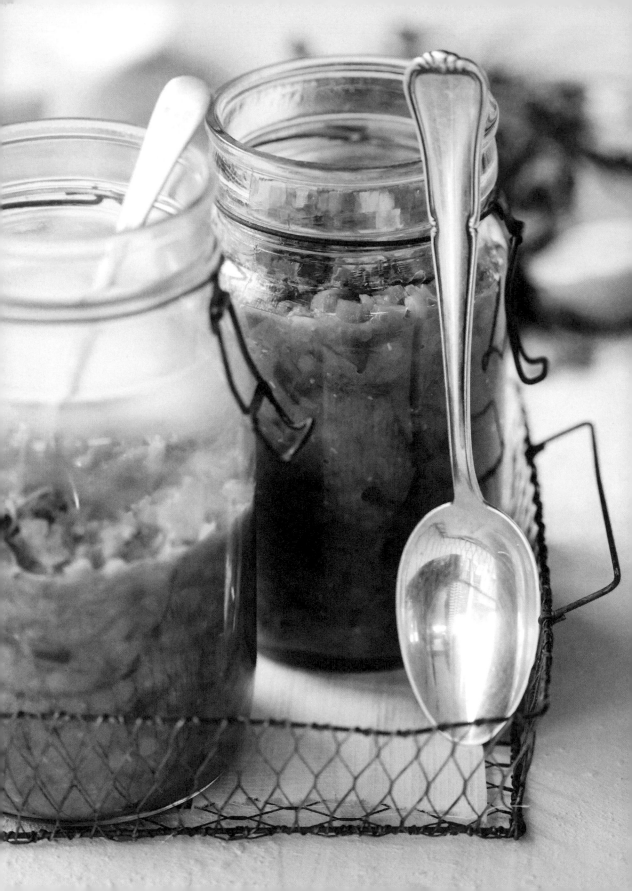

curried red lentil soup

1 tablespoon cold-pressed
extra-virgin coconut oil

1 small brown onion (100g),
chopped finely

2 cloves garlic, crushed

1 stalk celery (150g),
trimmed, chopped finely

1 medium carrot (120g), chopped finely

1 tablespoon mild curry powder

2 medium tomatoes (300g),
chopped finely

1 cup (200g) dried red lentils,
rinsed and drained

3 cups (750ml) filtered water

1 tablespoon tamari

2 medium green kale leaves
(80g), trimmed, shredded coarsely

1 tablespoon lime juice

¼ cup coarsely chopped
fresh flat-leaf parsley leaves

1 Heat oil in a medium saucepan; cook onion and garlic, stirring, until onion softens. Add celery and carrot; cook, stirring, 2 minutes or beginning to soften. Add curry powder; cook, stirring, 1 minute or until fragrant.

2 Add tomato, lentils, the water and tamari; bring to the boil. Reduce heat; simmer, covered, 10 minutes or until lentils are tender.

3 Stir kale and juice into soup. Season soup to taste; ladle into serving bowls. Serve topped with parsley.

prep + cook time 35 minutes
serves 2
nutritional count per serving protein (30.1g), carbohydrate (47.8g), total fat (12.1g), fibre (22.5g).

cook's notes

If you are taking this soup to work, pack the soup and the parsley separately. Reheat soup on the stovetop and serve topped with parsley. Soup will keep in an airtight container in the fridge for up to 3 days or freeze for up to 3 months.

"NEVER FORGET YOU ARE **TALENTED, BEAUTIFUL AND SIMPLY** THE BEST AT BEING **YOU.**"

DO THE CRAZY

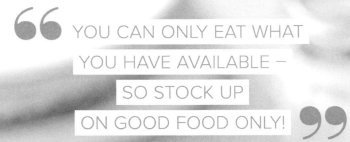

> YOU CAN ONLY EAT WHAT
> YOU HAVE AVAILABLE —
> SO STOCK UP
> ON GOOD FOOD ONLY!

roasted beetroot and lentil salad

4 baby golden beetroot (beets) (500g)

100g (3 ounces) swiss brown mushrooms, halved

1 teaspoon cold-pressed extra-virgin coconut oil

1 cup (200g) french-style fine green lentils

1 cup (50g) baby spinach leaves

½ cup loosely packed fresh flat-leaf parsley leaves

BALSAMIC AND HERB DRESSING

2 tablespoons balsamic vinegar

2 tablespoons cold-pressed extra-virgin coconut oil

1 tablespoon pure maple syrup

1 tablespoon coarsely chopped fresh chives

1 Preheat oven to 200°C/400°F.

2 Trim beetroot, leaving 5cm (2 inches) of the stems attached; reserve half the trimmed leaves for the salad; wash and drain well. Wrap beetroot individually in aluminium foil; place in a small baking dish. Roast about 30 minutes or until tender.

3 Combine mushrooms and oil in a small bowl; add to baking dish for last 5 minutes of beetroot cooking time.

4 Meanwhile, cook lentils in a medium saucepan of boiling filtered water, about 25 minutes or until tender. Drain.

5 When beetroot are cool enough to handle, peel them; cut into quarters or halves.

6 To make the balsamic and herb dressing, place ingredients in a screw-top jar, season to taste; shake well.

7 Combine beetroot, mushrooms, lentils, reserved beetroot leaves and parsley with the dressing in a large bowl; toss well to combine.

prep + cook time 50 minutes
serves 2
nutritional count per serving protein (33g), carbohydrate (55.1g), total fat (23.1g), fibre (20.7g).

cook's notes

If your beetroot leaves are not suitable for use in this salad, increase baby spinach leaves to 4 cups.

If you are taking this salad to work, pack salad and dressing separately. Keep salad in the fridge and dress just before serving. This salad would also be lovely sprinkled with some roasted pecans or walnuts and a little soft goat's cheese.

mexican fish and quinoa salad

¾ cup (150g) dried red quinoa

1 cup (250ml) filtered water

1 medium red capsicum (bell pepper) (200g), cut into 1cm (½-inch) pieces

3 yellow patty pan squash (90g), cut into 1cm (½-inch) pieces

1 baby eggplant (60g), cut into 1cm (½-inch) pieces

1 medium zucchini (120g), cut into 1cm (½-inch) pieces

½ small kumara (orange sweet potato) (100g), cut into 1cm (½-inch) pieces

1 small red onion (80g), cut into thin wedges

1 tablespoon cold-pressed extra-virgin coconut oil

2 teaspoons ground cumin

1 teaspoon hot paprika

2 x 150g (5-ounce) boneless, skinless snapper fillets

pinch ground cumin and hot paprika, extra

4 cups (120g) baby spinach leaves

LIME AND CORIANDER DRESSING

¼ cup (60ml) cold-pressed extra-virgin coconut oil

¼ cup (60ml) lime juice

2 tablespoons finely chopped fresh coriander (cilantro)

1 Preheat oven to 220°C/425°F.

2 Rinse quinoa well; drain. Place quinoa in a small saucepan with the water; stand 15 minutes. Bring to the boil. Reduce heat; cook quinoa, covered with a tight-fitting lid, about 15 minutes or until water is absorbed and quinoa is tender. Remove from heat; stand, covered, 10 minutes. Fluff with a fork.

3 Meanwhile, combine vegetables and onion with coconut oil and spices on a baking-paper-lined oven tray, season to taste; roast about 15 minutes or until browned and tender.

4 Place fish on another baking-paper-lined oven tray; sprinkle with extra spices, season. Roast, in oven, alongside vegetables, for last 10 minutes of vegetable cooking time or until cooked as desired.

5 To make the lime and coriander dressing, place ingredients in a screw-top jar, season to taste; shake well.

6 Combine quinoa, roasted vegetables, flaked fish and spinach with the dressing in a large bowl; toss well to combine.

prep + cook time 35 minutes (+ standing)
serves 2
nutritional count per serving protein (46.9g), carbohydrate (61.9g), total fat (44.4g), fibre (10.4g).

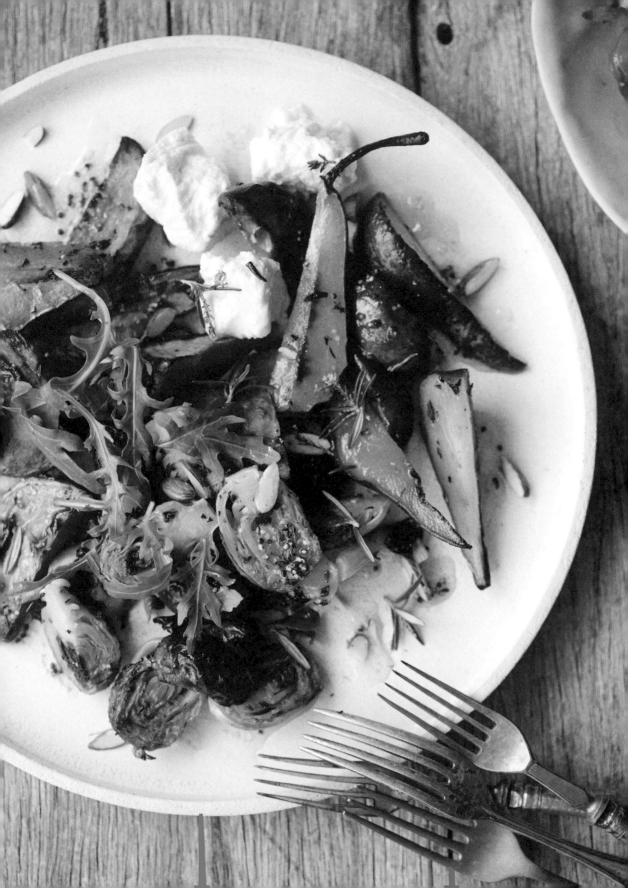

roasted pear, kumara and brussels sprout salad

1 large pear (330g)

½ medium kumara (orange sweet potato) (200g), chopped coarsely

250g (4 ounces) brussels sprouts, halved

2 teaspoons cold-pressed extra-virgin coconut oil

1 teaspoon finely chopped fresh rosemary leaves

3 cups (80g) baby rocket (arugula) leaves

¼ cup (40g) almond kernels, roasted, chopped coarsely

50g (1½ ounces) soft goat's cheese, crumbled

MACADAMIA AND MUSTARD DRESSING

2 tablespoons macadamia oil

2 tablespoons apple cider vinegar

1 teaspoon wholegrain mustard

1 teaspoon raw honey

1 Preheat oven to 200°C/400°F.

2 Cut unpeeled pear into 8 wedges; remove core. Combine pear, kumara and sprouts with the oil and rosemary in a small baking dish, season; roast about 25 minutes or until golden and tender.

3 To make the macadamia and mustard dressing, place ingredients in a screw-top jar, season to taste; shake well to combine.

4 Combine roasted pear, kumara and sprouts with rocket and the dressing in a large bowl; toss well to combine. Serve sprinkled with nuts and cheese.

prep + cook time 30 minutes
serves 2
nutritional count per serving protein (16.5g), carbohydrate (35.7g), total fat (40.3g), fibre (12.6g).

cook's notes

If you are taking this salad to work, pack salad and dressing separately. Keep salad in the fridge and dress just before serving.

You could add some poached chicken (see recipe on page 245) and toss it into the salad at Step 5.

----

kale, black rice and raspberry salad

1 cup (200g) black rice

150g (5 ounces) purple kale, trimmed, chopped coarsely

2 tablespoons cold-pressed extra-virgin coconut oil

½ cup (75g) fresh raspberries

½ cup (50g) roasted walnuts, chopped coarsely

50g (1½ ounces) soft goat's cheese, crumbled

RASPBERRY VINAIGRETTE

½ cup (75g) fresh raspberries

2 tablespoons cold-pressed extra-virgin coconut oil

1 tablespoon white wine vinegar

1 tablespoon filtered water

1 teaspoon raw honey

1 Rinse rice well; drain. Cook rice in a medium saucepan of boiling filtered water, about 25 minutes or until tender; drain. Rinse under cold water; drain.

2 Meanwhile, preheat oven to 200°C/400°F.

3 Combine kale with the oil on an oven tray, season; roast about 10 minutes or until crisp.

4 To make the raspberry vinaigrette, blend or process the ingredients until smooth and well combined.

5 Combine rice and kale with the vinaigrette in a large bowl; toss well to combine. Serve sprinkled with raspberries, nuts and cheese.

prep + cook time 35 minutes **serves** 2
nutritional count per serving protein (17.6g), carbohydrate (87.7g), total fat (52.6g), fibre (11.1g).

Kale is a true powerhouse vegie that is incredibly alkalizing, anti-inflammatory and rich in chlorophyll.

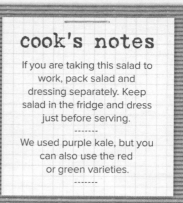

"THIS ONE DAY CANNOT BE EXCHANGED, REPLACED OR REFUNDED.

MAKE THE MOST OF IT

- LIVE ACTIVE. **"**

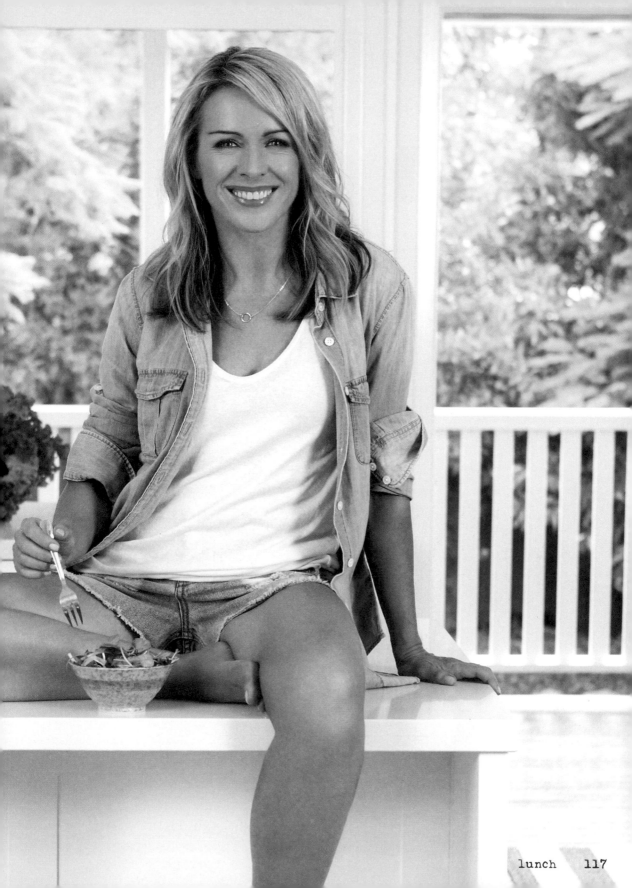

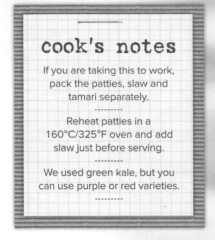

THAI FISH PATTIES WITH KALE, APPLE AND COCONUT SLAW

400g (12½ ounces) boneless skinless redfish fillets

1 tablespoon tamari

2 teaspoons fish sauce

1 clove garlic, quartered

1cm (½-inch) piece fresh ginger (5g), grated

½ small fresh thai red (serrano) chilli, chopped

½ cup loosely packed fresh coriander (cilantro) leaves

2 tablespoons sesame seeds

2 tablespoons tamari, extra

KALE, APPLE AND COCONUT SLAW

½ small fresh thai red (serrano) chilli, chopped finely

1 tablespoon unhulled tahini

1 tablespoon lime juice

1 tablespoon cold-pressed extra-virgin coconut oil

1 small apple (130g), cut into matchsticks (julienne)

1 cup finely shredded wombok (chinese/napa cabbage)

1 cup finely shredded green kale

½ cup firmly packed fresh mint leaves

½ cup (25g) flaked coconut

1 Process fish, tamari, fish sauce, garlic, ginger, chilli and coriander until combined. Using wet hands, shape mixture into 6 patties. Roll patties in sesame seeds.
2 Cook patties on a heated oiled grill plate (or grill or barbecue) about 2 minutes each side or until browned and cooked through.
3 Meanwhile, to make the kale, apple and coconut slaw, combine chilli, tahini, juice and oil in a medium bowl. Add the remaining ingredients; toss gently, season to taste.
4 Serve fish patties with slaw and extra tamari for dipping.

prep + cook time 40 minutes
serves 2
nutritional count per serving protein (53.4g), carbohydrate (13.9g), total fat (34.6g), fibre (7.7g).

Fish is packed with Omega-3 and is proven to help you live longer and actually make you smarter.

CHICKEN SANG CHOY BOW

cook's notes

If you are taking the sang choy bow to work, pack the chicken mixture, lettuce, coriander and nuts separately; keep refrigerated. Reheat the chicken mixture in a small frying pan and assemble in lettuce leaves just before serving. You could use lean minced (ground) turkey, beef or pork, instead of the chicken, for this recipe.

1 tablespoon sesame oil

1 small brown onion (100g), sliced thinly

400g (12½ ounces) minced (ground) chicken

2 cloves garlic, crushed

1 medium carrot (120g), grated coarsely

1 medium zucchini (120g), grated coarsely

1 cup finely shredded wombok (chinese/napa cabbage)

2 tablespoons tamari

1 tablespoon fish sauce

1 teaspoon finely grated lime rind

2 tablespoons lime juice

6 baby cos (romaine) lettuce leaves

⅓ cup loosely packed fresh coriander (cilantro) leaves

¼ cup (40g) coarsely chopped roasted unsalted cashews

1 Heat oil in a wok; stir-fry onion 2 minutes or until softened. Add chicken and garlic; stir-fry, 5 minutes or until chicken is browned, breaking up any large lumps.
2 Add carrot, zucchini, wombok, tamari and fish sauce; stir-fry until heated through. Remove from heat; stir in rind and juice.
3 Spoon chicken mixture into lettuce leaves; sprinkle with coriander and nuts.

prep + cook time 20 minutes
serves 2
nutritional count per serving protein (48.2g), carbohydrate (12.2g), total fat (35.9g), fibre (7g).

> " THIS DISH IS DEFINITELY WORTH GETTING YOUR HANDS DIRTY — BUT IF I'M EATING IT AT MY DESK, I SOMETIMES SHRED THE LETTUCE LEAVES AND THROW IT ALL IN A BOWL. "

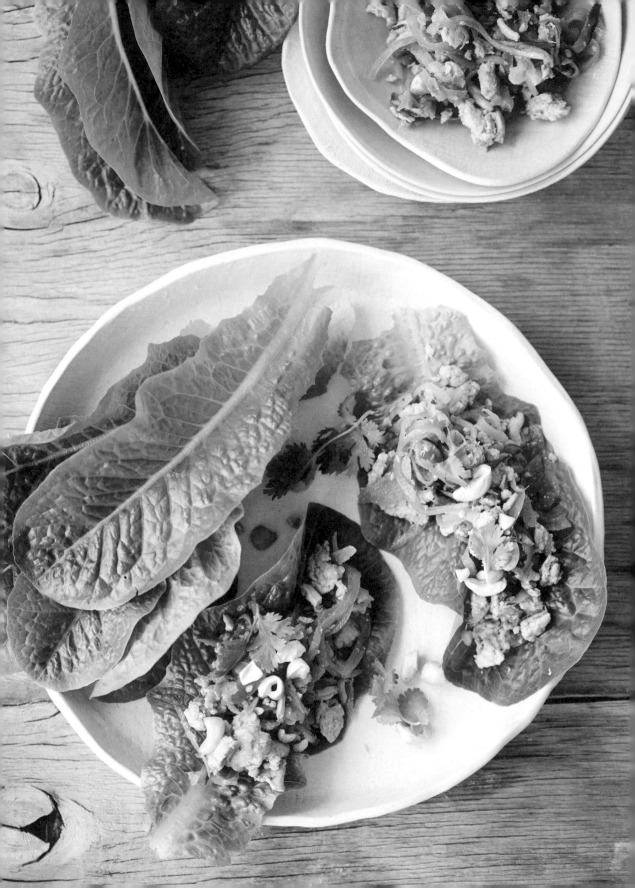

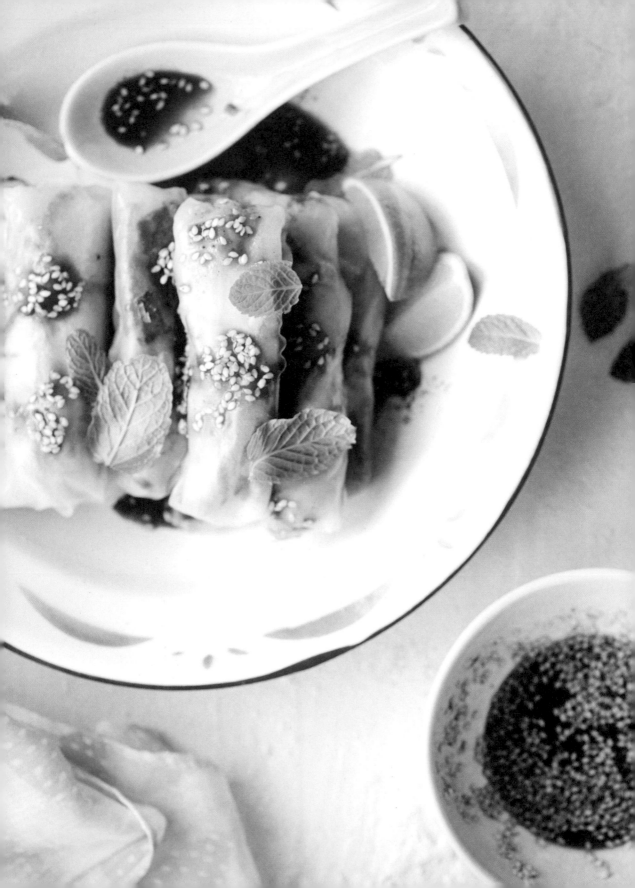

salmon, mint and cucumber rice paper rolls

200g (6½-ounce) boneless, skinless salmon fillet

2 teaspoons tamari

1 teaspoon sesame oil

½ teaspoon finely grated lime rind

6 x 22cm (9-inch) rice paper rounds

1 lebanese cucumber (130g), cut into thin matchsticks

6 small sprigs fresh mint leaves

1 Combine salmon, tamari, oil and rind in a small bowl; stand 10 minutes.
2 Cook salmon in a heated small non-stick frying pan about 5 minutes each side or until cooked as desired. Remove from heat; stand 5 minutes, then cut into 12 slices.
3 Dip one rice paper round into a bowl of warm water until soft. Lift sheet from water; place on a clean tea towel on bench. Top with 3-4 cucumber sticks, 2 salmon slices and a sprig of mint. Fold sheet over filling, then fold in both sides. Continue rolling to enclose filling.
4 Repeat step 3 to make a total of 6 rolls.
5 Serve rolls with tamarind and sesame dipping sauce (see recipe on this page).

prep + cook time 25 minutes
serves 2
nutritional count per serving (with dipping sauce) protein (39.2g), carbohydrate (71.6g), total fat (21g), fibre (2.4g).

tamarind and sesame dipping sauce

Combine 1 teaspoon tamarind puree, 2 tablespoons tamari, 1 teaspoon fish sauce, 1 tablespoon lime juice, 1 teaspoon sesame oil and 1 tablespoon toasted sesame seeds in a small bowl.

prep time 2 minutes
makes ⅓ cup (80ml)

This is also a great starter if you are having friends over for dinner.

thai-style vegetable rolls

6 large choy sum leaves (120g)

1 medium carrot (120g),
cut into thin matchsticks

1 small red capsicum (bell pepper)
(200g), cut into thin matchsticks

75g (2½ ounces) snow peas,
trimmed, sliced thinly lengthways

40g (1½ ounces) snow pea sprouts, trimmed

6 small sprigs fresh coriander (cilantro)

2 tablespoons finely chopped
roasted unsalted cashews

1 Trim and discard stems from choy
sum leaves.
2 Place one choy sum leaf on board, back-side
facing upwards. Press your finger along the rib
of the leaf to make leaf more pliable. Top with
some of the carrot, capsicum, snow pea and
snow pea sprouts; top with a sprig of
coriander, sprinkle with some of the nuts. Roll
choy sum leaf tightly around filling to enclose.
Place seam-side down on serving plate.
3 Repeat step 2 to make a total of 6 rolls.
4 Serve rolls with tamarind and sesame
dipping sauce (see recipe below).

prep time 25 minutes
serves 2
nutritional count per serving (with dipping
sauce) protein (12.1g), carbohydrate (11.9g),
total fat (12.6g), fibre (8.1g).

cook's notes

You can use collard greens, gai
lan leaves or some steamed
cabbage or silver beet (swiss
chard) leaves instead of the choy
sum leaves, if you prefer.

tamarind and sesame dipping sauce

Combine 1 teaspoon tamarind
puree, 2 tablespoons tamari,
1 teaspoon fish sauce, 1 tablespoon
lime juice, 1 teaspoon sesame oil
and 1 tablespoon toasted sesame
seeds in a small bowl.

prep time 2 minutes
makes ⅓ cup (80ml).

"FRESH FOOD LOADED WITH VITAMINS WILL GIVE YOU FAR MORE AMMUNITION AGAINST LINES, WRINKLES AND DRY SKIN THAN EXPENSIVE CREAMS."

gROW YOUR OWn

Food trends are just as seasonal as fashion trends (trust me, I know all about that!). And one trend that isn't going away any time soon is the REAL foods movement. We want our foods to be as fresh and close to nature as possible and what better way to be sure of this than to build a vegie patch and start growing some fruit and vegetables for yourself!

Aside from being rewarding and fun, growing your own produce provides fresh and nutritious food straight from the soil. And believe me, as soon as you start enjoying vegies direct from your own garden you'll never look back. You'll find that it changes the way you feel about food, and your body will begin to crave organic, nutritious, locally- or home-grown foods all of the time.

You can grow an edible garden anywhere you choose. It's simply about best using the space that you have, whether it's in a corner of your garden, moveable containers in your apartment, window boxes or pots of herbs in your kitchen.

GARDEN

Find out what fruits, vegetables and herbs grow best in your climate and space, decide on the best spot and get planting!

SOME IDEAS TO GET YOU STARTED:

* Start off small - you want your vegetable patch to be a labour of love, not an arduous chore!

* Think about how much you and your family eat, and try to grow your greens and other goodies in accordance with that (you don't want to grow too much of the same thing and end up wasting food!)

* Remember that some vegies, like tomato, cucumber and zucchini, will keep providing fruits throughout the season, which means you may not need as many plants as you think! Others, like carrots, radishes and corn only sprout once, so you might want to plant a few more of these.

* If you live in an apartment, consider growing herbs from a hanging pot, or on your windowsill! You may even be able to have a herb wall on your balcony.

4 essential dressings

Make every salad 'unforgettable' with these quick and easy homemade recipes.

LEMON DRESSING

HONEY MUSTARD
VINAIGRETTE

lemon dressing

- - - - - - - -

Combine ⅓ cup (80ml) lemon
juice, 4 drops natural stevia
liquid and pink Himalayan
salt and white pepper, to
taste in a screw-top jar;
shake well to combine.
prep time 5 minutes
makes ⅓ cup (80ml)

honey mustard vinaigrette

- - - - - - - - - -

Combine ¼ cup (60ml) cold-pressed
extra-virgin coconut oil, 1 tablespoon
apple cider vinegar, 1 teaspoon each raw
honey and dijon mustard, and pink
Himalayan salt and white pepper, to
taste, in a screw-top jar; shake well.
prep time 5 minutes
makes ½ cup (125ml)
note This recipe would also work well
with wholegrain mustard.

GREEN GODDESS
DRESSING

TAHINI AND ORANGE
DRESSING

green goddess dressing

Blend or process 1 cup loosely
packed fresh mint leaves, ½ cup
loosely packed fresh flat-leaf
parsley leaves, 1 teaspoon finely
grated lemon rind, 1½ tablespoons
lemon juice, 3 tablespoons cold-
pressed extra-virgin coconut oil
and pink Himalayan salt and white
pepper, to taste, until all herbs are
finely chopped. **prep time** 5
minutes **makes** ½ cup (125ml)

tahini and orange dressing

Combine ⅓ cup (80ml) orange
juice, 2 tablespoons tahini, 1
tablespoon cold-pressed
extra-virgin coconut oil (or filtered
water), 1 clove garlic, crushed, 2
teaspoons raw honey and pink
Himalayan salt and white pepper,
to taste, in a screw-top jar; shake
well. **prep time** 5 minutes
makes ½ cup (125ml)

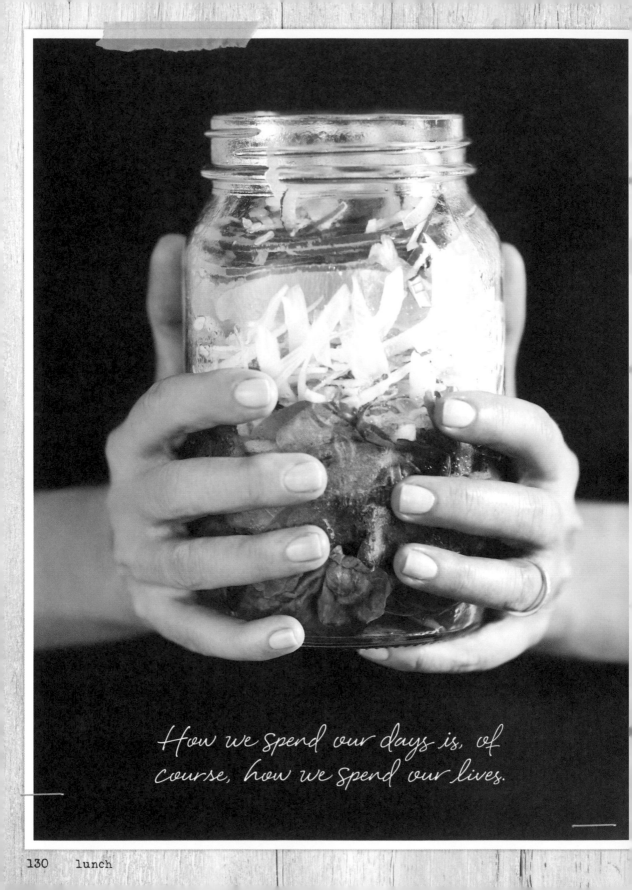

How we spend our days is, of course, how we spend our lives.

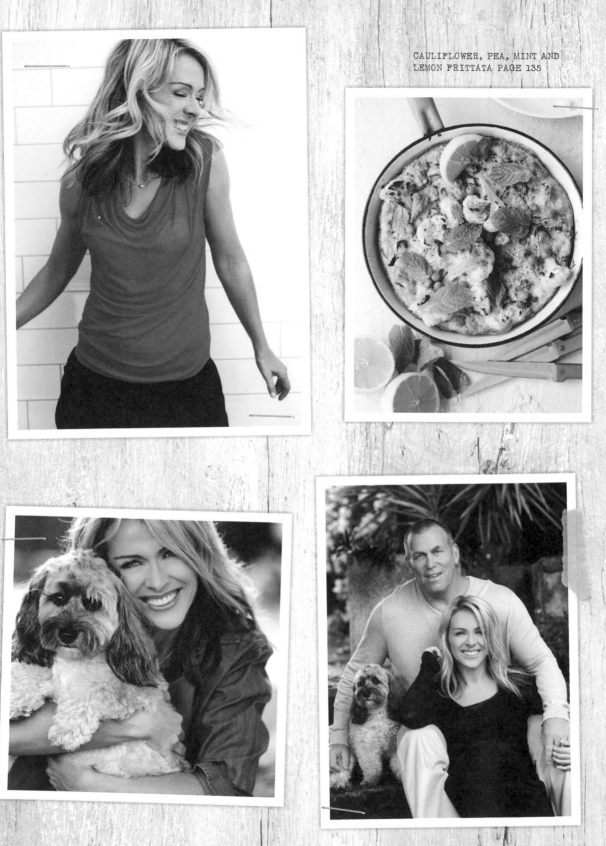

CAULIFLOWER, PEA, MINT AND
LEMON FRITTATA PAGE 135

frittata 3 ways

roasted kumara, asparagus and goat's cheese frittata

1 medium kumara (orange sweet potato) (400g), cut into 2cm (¾-inch) pieces

1 teaspoon cold-pressed extra-virgin coconut oil

1 small red onion (80g), sliced thinly

175g (5½ ounces) asparagus, trimmed, cut into 5cm (2-inch) lengths

1 tablespoon finely shredded fresh basil

6 organic free-range eggs

¼ cup (60ml) iced filtered water

50g (1½ ounces) soft goat's cheese, crumbled

1 Preheat oven to 200°C/400°F.

2 Place kumara on baking-paper-lined oven tray; drizzle with half the coconut oil. Roast about 30 minutes or until browned lightly and tender.

3 Heat remaining coconut oil in a small frying pan (top measurement about 20cm/8 inches); cook onion, stirring, until softened. Add asparagus; cook; stirring, about 3 minutes or until almost tender.

4 Add roasted kumara to pan; sprinkle with basil, toss gently. Whisk eggs and the water in a medium jug until frothy. Pour the egg mixture into pan; sprinkle with cheese. Cook frittata over medium-low heat, about 10 minutes or until about halfway set. Place pan in oven; cook frittata about 15 minutes or until browned and set.

5 Garnish with extra basil

prep + cook time 1 hour
serves 2
nutritional count per serving protein (29.7g), carbohydrate (28.1g), total fat (23.3g), fibre (5.2g).

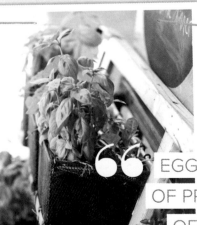

" EGGS PROVIDE AN ASTOUNDING 5G OF PROTEIN PER SERVE AND ARE ONE OF MY FAVOURITE BRAIN FOODS. "

cook's notes

For an interesting garnish, reserve some of the cooked vegetables and extra herbs to sprinkle over the cooked frittatas.

If you don't have an ovenproof frying pan, wrap the handle of your frying pan in aluminium foil to protect it from the heat of the oven.

QUINOA, MUSHROOM
AND SPINACH
FRITTATA

CAULIFLOWER, PEA,
MINT AND LEMON
FRITTATA

frittata 3 ways

quinoa, mushroom and spinach frittata

1 teaspoon cold-pressed extra-virgin coconut oil

200g (6½ ounces) swiss brown mushrooms, halved

2 cloves garlic, crushed

1 cup (50g) baby spinach leaves

¾ cup cooked white quinoa

6 organic free-range eggs

¼ cup (60ml) iced filtered water

1 Preheat oven to 200°C/400°F.
2 Heat coconut oil in a small frying pan (top measurement about 20cm/8 inches); cook mushrooms with garlic, stirring, until mushrooms are browned and tender.
3 Add spinach and quinoa to pan; toss gently. Whisk eggs and the water in a medium jug until frothy. Pour the egg mixture into pan; cook frittata over medium-low heat, about 10 minutes or until about halfway set. Place pan in oven; cook frittata about 15 minutes or until browned and set. Garnish with mushrooms and spinach leaves.

prep + cook time 40 minutes
serves 2
nutritional count per serving protein (25.7g), carbohydrate (14.9g), total fat (19.2g), fibre (4.5g).

cauliflower, pea, mint and lemon frittata

½ small cauliflower (500g), cut into florets

½ teaspoon cold-pressed extra-virgin coconut oil

¾ cup (90g) frozen peas

2 teaspoons finely grated lemon rind

1 tablespoon finely shredded fresh mint

6 organic free-range eggs

¼ cup (60ml) iced filtered water

1 Preheat oven to 200°C/400°F.
2 Steam cauliflower over a medium saucepan of simmering water, about 10 minutes or until just tender, drain.
3 Heat coconut oil in a small frying pan (top measurement about 20cm/8 inches); add cauliflower to pan with peas, toss gently. Sprinkle with rind and mint. Whisk eggs and the water in a medium jug until frothy. Pour the egg mixture into pan; cook frittata over medium-low heat, about 10 minutes or until about halfway set. Place pan in oven; cook frittata about 15 minutes or until browned and set. Garnish with florets, mint and cooked peas.

prep + cook time 45 minutes
serves 2
nutritional count per serving protein (27g), carbohydrate (9.7g), total fat (17.3g), fibre (10.5g).

lamb and mint patties with pomegranate and sunflower sprout salad

½ cup (100g) dried green lentils

250g (8 ounces) minced (ground) lamb

1 small red onion (80g), chopped finely

2 cloves garlic, crushed

1 tablespoon tamari

2 tablespoons finely chopped fresh mint

1 teaspoon each ground coriander and ground cumin

POMEGRANATE AND SUNFLOWER SPROUT SALAD

1 large carrot (180g)

1 lebanese cucumber (130g)

⅓ cup (80ml) pomegranate pulp (juice and seeds)

1 tablespoon cold-pressed extra-virgin coconut oil

1 tablespoon red wine vinegar

1 clove garlic, crushed

1 teaspoon raw honey

2 cups (60g) sunflower sprouts

½ cup firmly packed fresh mint leaves

1 Rinse lentils well; drain. Cook lentils in a small saucepan of boiling filtered water about 15 minutes or until tender; drain. Rinse under cold water; drain.
2 Combine lamb, lentils, onion, garlic, tamari, mint and spices in a medium bowl. Shape mixture into 6 patties.
3 Cook patties on a heated oiled grill plate (or grill or barbecue) about 2 minutes each side or until browned and cooked through.
4 Meanwhile, to make the pomegranate and sunflower sprout salad, use a vegetable peeler to slice carrot and cucumber into long thin ribbons. Whisk the pomegranate, oil, vinegar, garlic and honey in a medium bowl until combined. Add the carrot, cucumber, sprouts and mint; toss gently, season to taste.
5 Serve lamb patties with salad.

prep + cook time 40 minutes
serves 2
nutritional count per serving protein (44.2g), carbohydrate (36.3g), total fat (28.1g), fibre (16.8g).

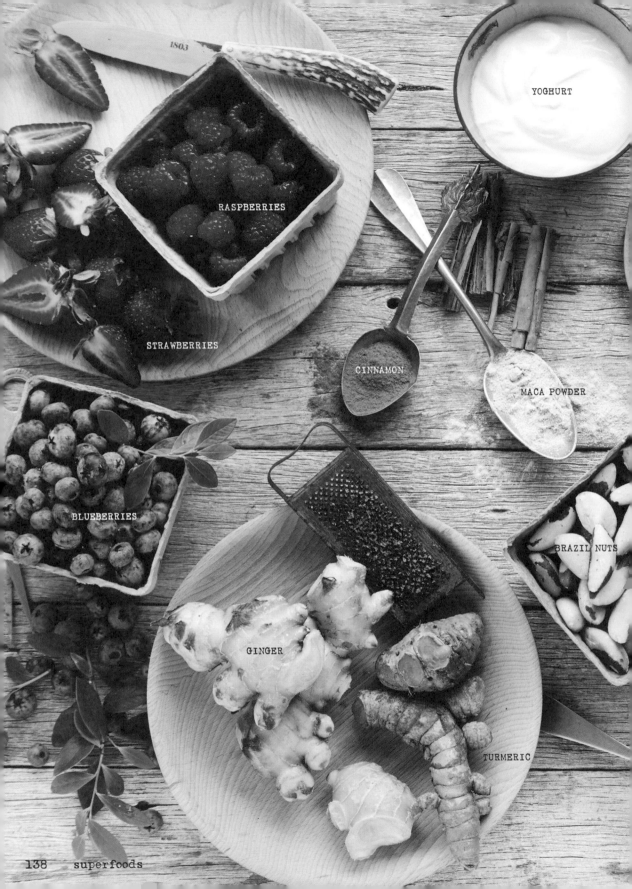

YOGHURT

RASPBERRIES

STRAWBERRIES

CINNAMON

MACA POWDER

BLUEBERRIES

BRAZIL NUTS

GINGER

TURMERIC

SALMON

WHITE CHIA
SEEDS

ACAI

BLACK CHIA
SEEDS

SUPERFOODS

Superfoods are here
to stay; and these are
just some of the super
ingredients that have
honestly changed my
life! Not only do they
taste delicious but these
powerhouse foods are
packed with nutrients and
antioxidants and I try to
use a mix of them in the
food I eat every day.

BEE POLLEN

TOMATOES

COCONUT OIL

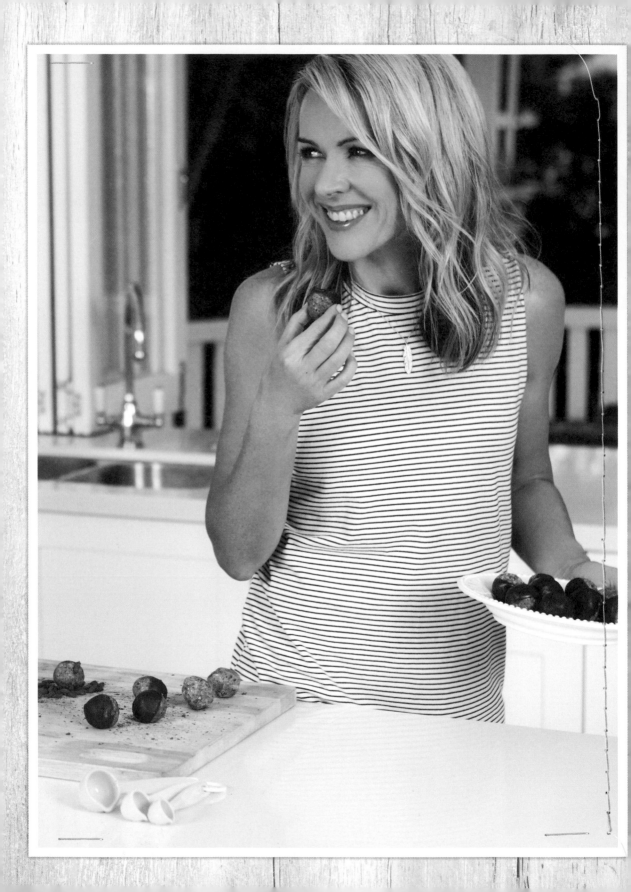

SNACKS

Having a few REAL food, nutrient-rich snacks between meals is a wonderful way to keep your metabolism going and in my opinion, absolutely essential to ward off mid-morning or afternoon junk food cravings.

In fact, snacks are an integral part of my daily food plan. They keep my blood sugar at an even level, keep my mind sharp and help maintain my metabolism at a healthy speed.

Snacks are there for the times when you get hungry between meals and I always check myself when reaching for them - to make sure I am actually hungry and not just thirsty, or bored! It's important to have snacks to hand, but equally important that you don't just eat them because they are there.

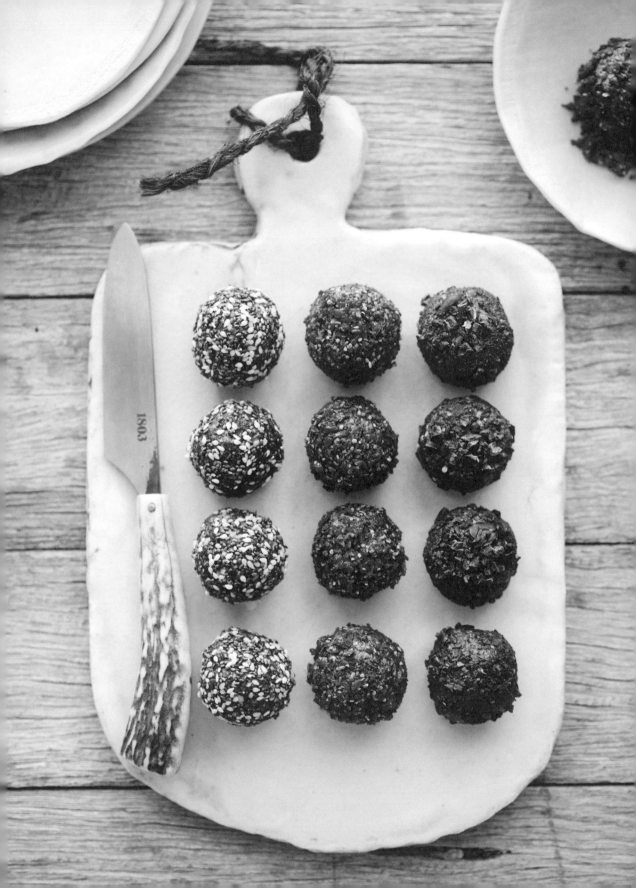

honey and sesame spirulina balls

1 cup (140g) macadamias

1 cup (150g) cashews

½ cup (40g) desiccated coconut

⅓ cup (90g) unhulled tahini

⅓ cup (115g) raw honey

1 tablespoon spirulina powder

1 teaspoon vanilla bean paste

2 tablespoons sesame seeds

2 tablespoons black chia seeds

1 Process nuts, coconut, tahini, honey, spirulina and vanilla until combined.
2 Roll level tablespoons of mixture into balls. Roll balls in combined sesame seeds and chia seeds, place on baking-paper-lined tray; refrigerate or freeze 30 minutes or until firm.

prep time 25 minutes (+ refrigeration or freezing) **makes** 20 balls
nutritional count per ball protein (4g), carbohydrate (7.3g), total fat (14.3g), fibre (1.8g).

cook's notes

Spirulina balls can be refrigerated, in an airtight container, for up to 4 days or freeze them for up to 3 months.

You can roll these balls in whatever coatings you like. Try a combination of 1 tablespoon finely chopped goji berries and 1 tablespoon fine desiccated coconut. You can also roll in cacao nibs.

" *In-between meals is often when we fall off the wagon, so making sure we have healthy snacks on hand is important* "

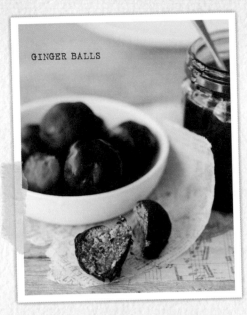

GINGER BALLS

ginger balls

1 cup (140g) macadamias

½ cup (70g) shelled pistachios

6 fresh dates (120g), seeded, chopped coarsely

1cm (½-inch) piece fresh ginger (5g), grated

4 tablespoons finely chopped cacao butter

½ cup (50g) cacao powder

2 teaspoons coconut sugar

1 Process nuts, dates and ginger until mixture forms a coarse, rollable dough.
2 Roll level tablespoons of the mixture into balls. Place on baking-paper-lined tray; refrigerate or freeze 30 minutes or until firm.
3 Meanwhile, stir cacao butter in a small heatproof bowl over a small saucepan of simmering water; remove from heat, stir in sifted cacao powder and sugar until smooth.
4 Coat each ball in cacao mixture. Return to tray; freeze until chocolate sets.

prep time 25 minutes (+ refrigeration or freezing) **makes** 14 balls
nutritional count per ball protein (2.9g), carbohydrate (7.8g), total fat (14.1g), fibre (1.8g).

cacao, chia and hazelnut protein balls

1½ cups (210g) hazelnuts

1 cup (170g) dried seeded prunes

½ cup (40g) desiccated coconut

⅓ cup (35g) natural wholegrain brown rice protein powder

2 tablespoons pure maple syrup

1 tablespoon cacao powder

1 tablespoon black chia seeds

2 tablespoons cacao powder, extra

1 Process nuts, prunes, coconut, protein powder, maple syrup, cacao powder and chia seeds until combined.
2 Roll level tablespoons of mixture into balls. Roll balls in extra cacao powder, place on baking-paper-lined tray; refrigerate or freeze 1 hour or until firm.

prep time 25 minutes (+ refrigeration or freezing) **makes** 14 balls
nutritional count per ball protein (3.7g), carbohydrate (10.8g), total fat (11.8g), fibre (3.2g).

THESE SNACKS ARE ALL-ROUND WINNERS AND I FREEZE THEM SO I'M NOT TEMPTED TO EAT THEM ALL AT ONCE!

CACAO, CHIA AND
HAZELNUT PROTEIN BALLS

These are the perfect snack, dessert or gift.

DIPS

See following pages for recipes

SPINACH HUMM

LEMON AND THYME
CARROT DIP

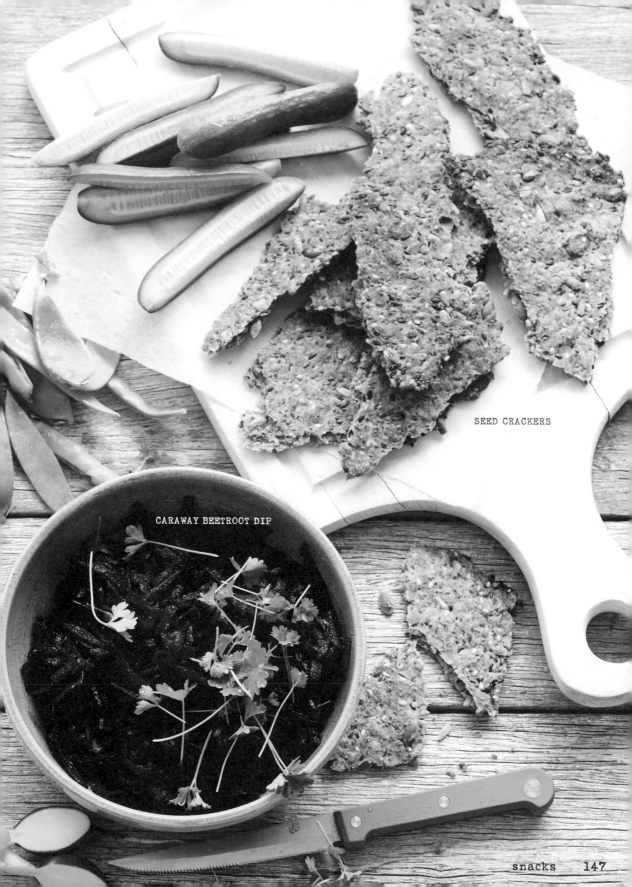

SEED CRACKERS

CARAWAY BEETROOT DIP

DIPS

lemon and thyme carrot dip

3 medium carrots (360g), chopped coarsely

2 cloves garlic, peeled

4 sprigs fresh thyme

5cm (2-inch) strip lemon rind

1 tablespoon lemon juice

1 Cook carrot with garlic, thyme and rind in a small saucepan of boiling water about 15 minutes or until carrot is tender. Drain. Discard thyme and rind.

2 Blend or process carrot and garlic with juice until smooth; season to taste. Sprinkle with 2 teaspoons of chopped pistachios if you like. Serve with vegetable sticks or seed crackers (see recipe opposite).

prep + cook time 20 minutes
makes 1½ cups
nutritional count per ¼ cup protein (0.5g), carbohydrate (2.8g), total fat (0.1g), fibre (2.2g).

caraway beetroot dip

½ teaspoon caraway seeds

2 medium beetroot (beets) (350g), trimmed, peeled, grated coarsely

1 tablespoon finely chopped fresh flat-leaf parsley

2 tablespoons apple cider vinegar

1 teaspoon pure maple syrup

1 teaspoon wholegrain mustard

1 Dry-fry seeds in a small frying pan over low heat until fragrant. Cool.

2 Combine caraway with remaining ingredients in a small bowl; season to taste. Sprinkle with 2 teaspoons microherbs, if you like. Serve with vegetable sticks or seed crackers (see recipe opposite).

prep + cook time 20 minutes
makes 1½ cups
nutritional count per ¼ cup protein (0.8g), carbohydrate (4.1g), total fat (0.1g), fibre (1.6g).

cook's notes

These dips will keep in an airtight container in the fridge for up to 3 days. Seed crackers will keep in an airtight container for up to 1 week.

seed crackers

2 tablespoons black chia seeds

2 tablespoons linseeds

½ cup (125ml) warm water

1¼ cups (200g) wholemeal spelt flour

1 teaspoon sea salt flakes

⅓ cup (65g) pepitas (pumpkin seeds)

⅓ cup (50g) sunflower seed kernels

2 tablespoons sesame seeds

1 organic free-range egg

⅓ cup (80g) cold-pressed
extra-virgin coconut oil

1 Preheat oven to 200°C/400°F.
2 Combine chia seeds, linseeds and the
water in a medium bowl; stand 20 minutes,
stirring occasionally.
3 Add flour, salt, pepitas, sunflower seeds,
sesame seeds, egg and oil; mix with hands
until well combined. Divide dough in half.
4 Roll each portion of dough between
sheets of baking paper until 20cm x 30cm
(8-inch x 12-inch) rectangle, 5mm (¼-inch)
thick. Slide each paper onto an oven tray;
remove top papers.
5 Bake crackers about 25 minutes or until
lightly browned and crisp. Cool on trays before
breaking into pieces.

prep + cook time 40 minutes
(+ standing) **makes** approximately
50 pieces
nutritional count per per piece protein (1.6g),
carbohydrate (2.5g), total fat (3.3g), fibre (0.3g).

spinach hummus

½ cup (100g) dried chickpeas
(garbanzo beans)

80g (2½ ounces) baby spinach leaves

1 clove garlic, quartered

2 tablespoons tahini

2 tablespoons lemon juice

1 tablespoon water

pinch cayenne pepper

1 Place chickpeas in a small bowl, cover
with cold water; stand overnight. Drain.
2 Cook chickpeas in a small saucepan of
boiling water about 20 minutes or until
tender. Add spinach to pan; stir until spinach
is wilted. Drain.
3 Blend or process chickpeas and spinach
with remaining ingredients until smooth;
season to taste. Serve with vegetable sticks
or seed crackers.

prep + cook time 25 minutes (+ standing)
makes 1½ cups
nutritional count per ¼ cup protein (7.1g),
carbohydrate (2.6g), total fat (7.5g), fibre (4.3g).

tamari and honey nut nibbles

1 tablespoon tamari

2 teaspoons raw honey

½ cup (70g) macadamias

½ cup (80g) brazil nuts

½ cup (50g) walnuts

½ cup (80g) almond kernels

½ cup (75g) cashews

¼ cup (50g) pepitas (pumpkin seeds)

¼ cup (35g) sunflower seeds

cook's notes

I freeze these nuts and just defrost them as I need them. If you would prefer a sweeter version of this recipe, omit the tamari and add 2 teaspoons ground cinnamon to the honey mixture.

----

1 Preheat oven to 180°C/350°F. Line an oven tray with baking paper.
2 Bring tamari and honey to the boil in a small saucepan, stirring. Remove from heat; stir in nuts and seeds, mix well.
3 Spread nut mixture onto oven tray; bake about 10 minutes or until browned and crisp, stirring occasionally. Cool on tray, stirring occasionally.

prep + cook time 20 minutes (+ cooling)
makes 3 cups (6 x ½-cup serves)
nutritional count per ½ cup protein (14.4g), carbohydrate (7.2g), total fat (42g), fibre (3.7g).

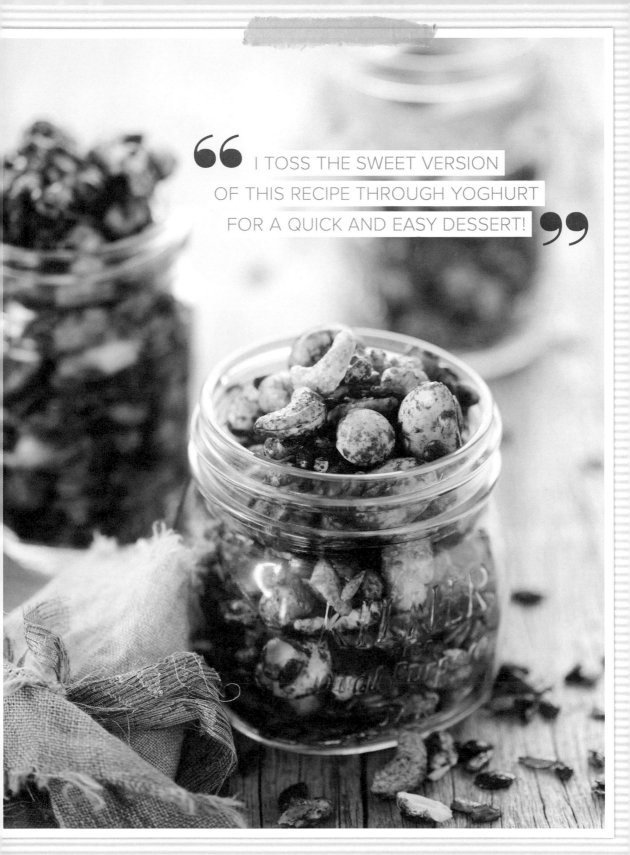

" I TOSS THE SWEET VERSION OF THIS RECIPE THROUGH YOGHURT FOR A QUICK AND EASY DESSERT! "

VEGIE STICKS
WITH NUT BUTTER
FOR RECIPE, SEE PAGE 164

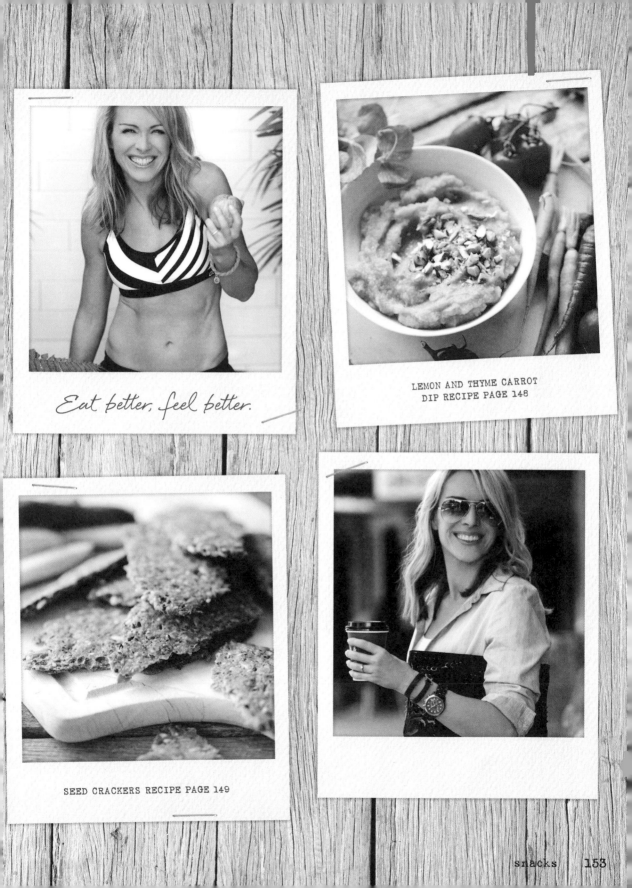

Eat better, feel better.

LEMON AND THYME CARROT
DIP RECIPE PAGE 148

SEED CRACKERS RECIPE PAGE 149

"MUNG BEANS ARE PACKED
WITH NUTRIENTS THAT HELP CLEANSE
YOUR DIGESTION AND BOOST
YOUR METABOLISM."

CHICKEN AND MUNG BEAN MEATLOAF MUFFINS

²/₃ cup (135g) dried mung beans

600g (1¼ pounds) minced (ground) chicken

2 organic free-range eggs

1 clove garlic, crushed

1 medium brown onion (150g), grated

1 medium carrot (120g), grated

1 medium zucchini (120g), grated

1 medium red capsicum (bell pepper) (200g), chopped finely

2 teaspoons ground cumin

1 teaspoon ground turmeric

2 tablespoons each finely chopped fresh basil and flat-leaf parsley

1 Place beans in a medium bowl, cover with cold water; stand overnight; drain.
2 Place beans in a medium saucepan, cover with cold water, bring to a boil and cook about 20 minutes or until tender; drain. Rinse under cold water; drain.
3 Meanwhile, preheat oven to 180°C/350°F.
4 Combine beans with remaining ingredients in a large bowl; season. Line 12-hole (⅓-cup/80ml) standard muffin pan with squares of baking paper. Divide mixture evenly into each hole.
5 Bake meatloaf muffins about 30 minutes or until browned and cooked through. Cool muffins in pan for 5 minutes. Garnish with parsley leaves, if you like.

prep + cook time 1 hour (+ standing)
makes 12
nutritional count per muffin protein (14.1g), carbohydrate (6.5g), total fat (5.2g), fibre (4.2g).

cook's notes
You can make your own tomato sauce to serve with these muffins by blending 4 seeded and coarsely chopped ripe tomatoes with 1 tablespoon of tamari and balsamic vinegar until smooth.

CHOC-CRUNCH BANANAS

⅓ cup (50g) finely chopped cacao butter

2 tablespoons cacao powder

1 tablespoon pure maple syrup

3 medium bananas (600g)

½ cup (80g) finely chopped goji berries

½ cup (25g) toasted shredded coconut

1 Stir cacao butter in a small heatproof bowl set over a small saucepan of simmering water until melted (do not let base of bowl touch the water). Remove from heat; whisk in sifted cacao powder and maple syrup until smooth.

2 Cut each banana in half; push onto paddle pop sticks. Dip banana into cacao mixture, drain off excess; place on baking-paper-lined tray. Freeze about 5 minutes or until set.

3 Combine berries and coconut. Dip banana into cacao mixture again, drain off excess. Dip in coconut mixture to coat. Place on baking-paper-lined tray. Freeze about 5 minutes or until set.

prep + cook time 25 minutes
(+ freezing) **makes** 6
nutritional count per piece protein (2.3g), carbohydrate (18.4g), total fat (11.5g), fibre (1.7g).

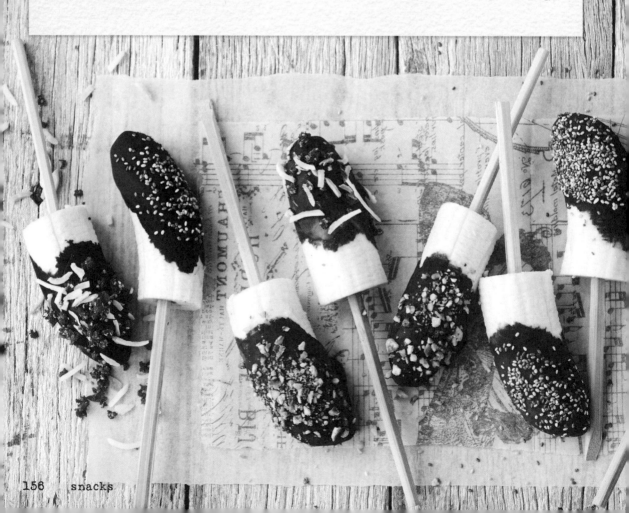

variations

1. Replace berries and coconut with 1 cup (160g) finely chopped pistachios

------

2. Replace berries and coconut with ½ cup (80g) white and black chia seeds

------

cook's notes

Bananas will keep, in an airtight container in the freezer for up to 3 months; that's if you haven't eaten them all by then!

MYTH BUSTERS

WITH SO MANY MYTHS FLOATING AROUND ABOUT HEALTHY FOODS AND HEALTHY EATING, I THOUGHT I'D PICK OUT A FEW OF THE MORE COMMON ONES AND SET THE RECORD STRAIGHT. THAT WAY, YOU WON'T GET FOOLED INTO THINKING SOME UNHEALTHY AND POTENTIALLY DANGEROUS FOOD PRACTICES ARE ACTUALLY GOOD FOR YOU!

MYTH: EATING LESS IS BETTER

FACT: All eating less does is slow down your metabolism and make your body store more fat. Eating smaller meals more frequently and ensuring they are comprised of healthy, nutritious REAL foods, is the only way to stay healthy and maintain your ideal weight.

MYTH: YOU NEED TO AVOID CARBS

FACT: Your body NEEDS carbs to function. Just choose your carbs wisely. Avoid processed and simple carbs (think white potatoes, white bread, white pasta) and instead choose complex carbs that deliver energy slowly and steadily. Think wholegrains like quinoa, wholemeal pasta, sweet potato and rice.

MYTH: ENERGY DRINKS ARE GOOD

FACT: Oh, this myth frustrates me more than most! Energy drinks are NOT good. Neither is vitamin water. They are loaded with refined, processed sugar and loads of artificial flavours and colours. If you want a REAL energy drink – try a green smoothie, coconut water or juice!

MYTH: SUGAR IS THE ENEMY

FACT: Sugar, in its natural, unrefined and unprocessed form, is actually good for you – in moderation. If you want a sugar replacement that is all natural, turn to page 204 to read about my favourites.

MYTH: LOW FAT IS BEST

FACT: Low fat usually means highly processed and filled with chemicals. Low fat can also leave you feeling unsatisfied, and make you reach for other, less healthy foods later on. As always, I suggest consuming food as close to its natural form as possible, and if that means a higher fat content, then be wise about your portion size!

MYTH: BOTTLED WATER IS BEST

FACT: Bottled water can sometimes be filled with harmful chemicals, which leach out of the plastic and into the water, especially when exposed to heat or sunlight. These chemicals have been linked to cancer and other diseases. It also takes a great deal of energy to produce bottled water, which makes our carbon footprint even greater. The best solution is to buy yourself a water filter and filter the water from your tap.

MYTH: YOU MUST HAVE DAIRY

FACT: We have been led to believe that we need dairy every day to keep our calcium levels high and our bones strong. The truth is that you can find rich sources of calcium in the plant-based foods you eat. Green leafy vegetables such as broccoli, spinach and Asian greens are packed full of calcium, as are kale, kidney beans, tofu, wholegrains and nuts.

MYTH: I CAN GET ENOUGH VITAMIN D FROM MY FOOD

FACT: It is almost impossible to have your entire vitamin D requirements met by food, as much as I hate to admit it. The body requires vitamin D for bone strength and immunity and the best source of vitamin D is 15 minutes of unprotected sunlight exposure each day. Now, don't think you can go out in the middle of the day and blitz it – you'll just put yourself at risk of sunburn and skin cancer. Instead, get up as the sun is rising and walk for one hour in the morning light. This will do the trick! Team it with lots of vitamin D rich foods, like fatty wild fish (not farmed), free-range, organic whole eggs and shiitake mushrooms.

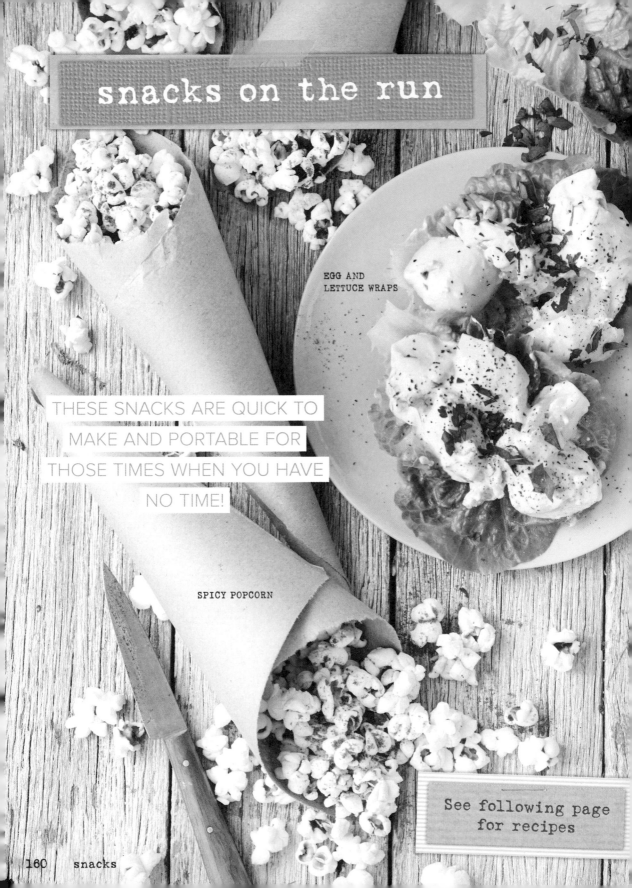

snacks on the run

EGG AND
LETTUCE WRAPS

THESE SNACKS ARE QUICK TO MAKE AND PORTABLE FOR THOSE TIMES WHEN YOU HAVE NO TIME!

SPICY POPCORN

See following page for recipes

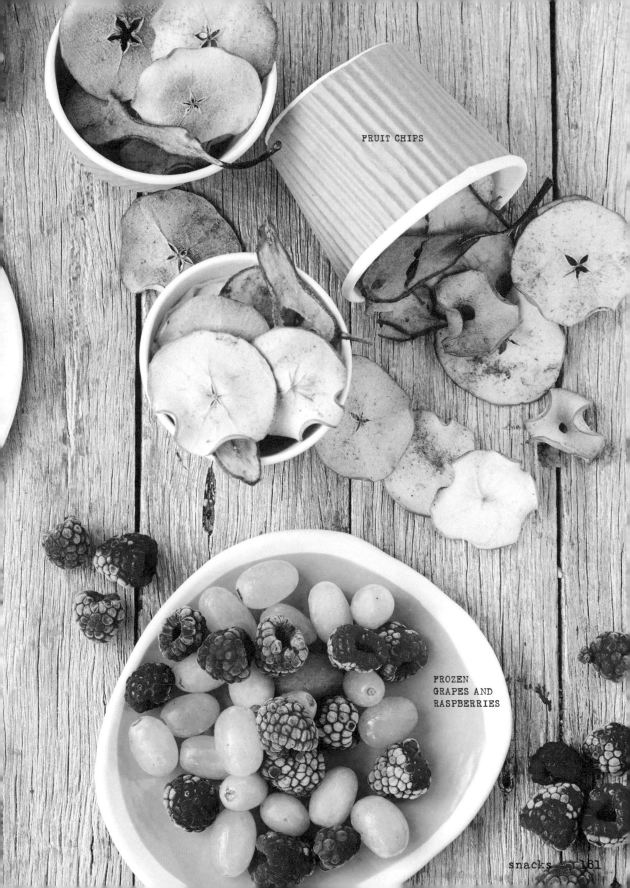

FRUIT CHIPS

FROZEN
GRAPES AND
RASPBERRIES

snacks on the run

spicy popcorn

Place 2 tablespoons popping corn into a medium saucepan; cover with a tight-fitting lid. Turn the heat to high and wait for the popping to start. Turn off the heat and wait for the popping to stop before removing the lid. While popcorn is still warm, quickly and carefully toss in ½ teaspoon each of ground cumin and ground cinnamon and a pinch of ground cayenne pepper.

----

prep + cook time 10 minutes
serves 2 (makes 2 cups)
nutritional count per serving protein (1.9g), carbohydrate (13.3g), total fat (0.9g), fibre (0g).

egg and lettuce wraps

With a fork, roughly mash 4 hard-boiled organic free-range eggs together with ¼ cup (70g) greek yoghurt and 2 teaspoons dijon mustard in a small bowl. Stir in 2 teaspoons finely chopped fresh flat-leaf parsley. Season to taste. Serve egg mixture in 4 baby cos (romaine) lettuce leaves.

----

prep time 10 minutes **serves** 2
nutritional count per serving protein (16.9g), carbohydrate (19.9g), total fat (13.5g), fibre (0.5g).

fruit chips

Preheat oven to 120°C/250°F. Using a
mandoline or v-slicer, slice 1 medium apple
(150g) crossways into thin rounds; slice 1
medium firm pear (230g) thinly lengthways.
Discard any seeds from fruit slices. Using
hands, carefully toss fruit slices with 2
teaspoons pure maple syrup and ½ teaspoon
mixed spice in a medium bowl to coat. Place
fruit slices, in single layer, on wire racks over
oven trays. Bake about 1 hour 10 minutes or
until dried and crisp. Cool.

----

prep + cook time 1 hour 45 minutes **serves** 2
nutritional count per serving protein (0.6g),
carbohydrate (26.8g), total fat (0.2g), fibre (4.1g).

frozen grapes and raspberries

Freeze 1 cup (175g) seedless green grapes
and 1 cup (150g) raspberries about
3 hours or until firm.

----

prep time 5 minutes (+ freezing)
serves 2
nutritional count per serving protein
(1.4g), carbohydrate (18.7g), total fat (0.3g),
fibre (5.4g).

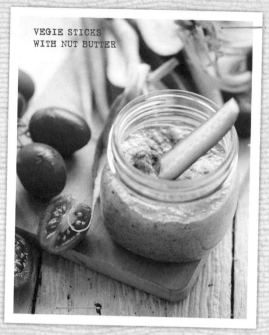

VEGIE STICKS
WITH NUT BUTTER

coconut yoghurt
with mixed berries

Combine 1½ cups coconut yoghurt (see recipe
on page 60) 2 teaspoons acai powder,
2 teaspoons white chia seeds and 1 teaspoon
bee pollen in a small bowl.
Serve yoghurt mixture with 1 cup (125g) mixed
berries. To serve, sprinkle with another
1 teaspoon bee pollen.

- -

prep time 5 minutes **serves** 2
nutritional count per serving protein (5.6g),
carbohydrate (17.8g), total fat (35.9g), fibre (1g).

vegie sticks
with nut butter

Cut 2 stalks celery (300g) and 1 large carrot (180g)
into matchsticks; serve with ½ cup (140g) natural
almond butter (or your favourite natural nut butter).

- -

prep time 5 minutes **serves** 2
nutritional count per serving including vegie sticks
protein (14.4g), carbohydrate (8.1g), total fat (38g),
fibre (3.9g).

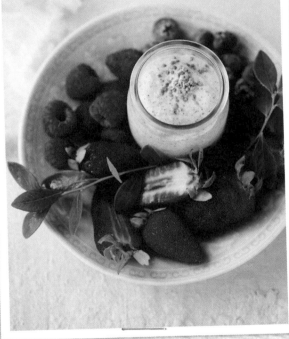

COCONUT YOGHURT
WITH MIXED BERRIES

cook's notes

You can use any vegies you like,
such as cherry tomatoes,
radishes or cucumber.

- - - - - - - - - -

Try making your own nut butter –
roast unsalted nuts (about 4 cups
will make a small jar of nut butter)
until browned lightly. Cool;
process about 3 minutes, or until
mixture forms a coarse paste,
scraping down sides occasionally.
Add Himalayan pink salt to taste.
Process again about 3 minutes
or until smooth.

- - - - - - - - - -

YOGHURT
IS A POWERHOUSE
TO IMPROVE IMMUNITY AND
DIGESTIVE HEALTH.

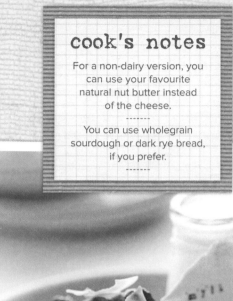

COTTAGE CHEESE AND
MIXED BERRIES ON TOAST

cottage cheese and mixed berries on toast

Combine 1 cup (125g) mixed berries and 2 tablespoons orange juice in a small bowl; refrigerate about 10 minutes or until berries begin to soften. Toast 2 slices MNB seed and nut bread (see page 240); spread with ⅓ cup (65g) cottage cheese, top with berry mixture. Sprinkle with 1 tablespoon toasted flaked coconut, toasted rolled oats, or pinch of cinnamon, if you like.

prep time 5 minutes **serves** 2
nutritional count per serving protein (16.6g), carbohydrate (16.6g), total fat (23.2g), fibre (4.3g).

avocado with lemon and herbs

Cut 1 medium avocado (250g) into quarters; discard seed. Serve avocado drizzled with 2 tablespoons lemon juice. Sprinkle with 2 teaspoons finely chopped coriander (cilantro) or parsley.

prep time 5 minutes **serves** 2
nutritional count per serving protein (2.1g), carbohydrate (1g), total fat (20.2g), fibre (2.8g).

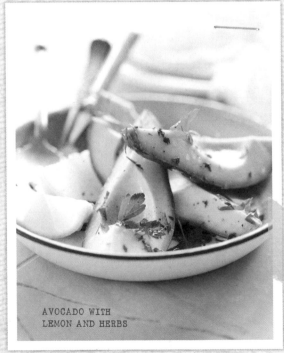

AVOCADO WITH
LEMON AND HERBS

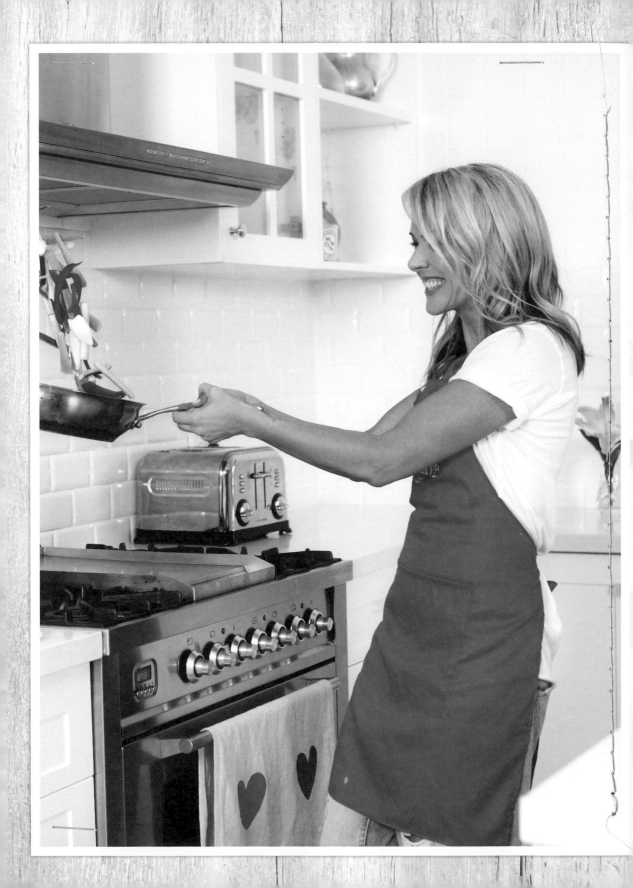

DINNER

Nothing makes me happier than sitting down to a meal with family and friends, and what better way to share your day and unforgettable moments than over lovingly prepared, nutritious and delicious food.

As the final meal of the day, dinner is also the perfect opportunity to balance out your nutrient intake, and this section contains many of the meals you could expect at my dining room table most nights. They are all pretty simple to make, satisfying without overloading your digestive system and contain a variety of nutrients guaranteed to end your day on a delicious high-note every time.

I'm sure you will find them easy to create and I hope you enjoy them enough to make them your favourites too.

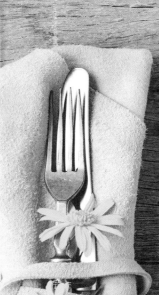

CHILLI AND GARLIC PRAWN SKEWERS WITH QUINOA AND CAULIFLOWER PILAF

12 uncooked medium king prawns (shrimp) (540g)

½ fresh small red thai (serrano) chilli, chopped finely

2 cloves garlic, crushed

2 teaspoons finely grated lime rind

1 teaspoon finely chopped fresh coriander (cilantro) root and stem mixture

1 tablespoon cold-pressed extra-virgin coconut oil

1 lime, cut into wedges

QUINOA PILAF

¾ cup (150g) dried red quinoa

1 teaspoon cold-pressed extra-virgin coconut oil

1 small red onion (100g), sliced thinly

1 clove garlic, crushed

1 teaspoon each ground cumin and coriander

½ small cauliflower (500g), cut into small florets

1¼ cups (310ml) filtered water

3 medium kale leaves (120g), trimmed, shredded coarsely

2 tablespoons roasted slivered almonds

½ cup loosely packed fresh coriander (cilantro) leaves

1 Shell and devein prawns, leaving tails intact. Combine prawns, chilli, garlic, rind, coriander root and stem mixture and oil in a medium bowl; toss well to combine. Cover; refrigerate 30 minutes.

2 Meanwhile, to make the quinoa pilaf, rinse quinoa well; drain. Heat oil in a small saucepan; cook, onion, garlic and spices, stirring, until onion softens. Add quinoa, cauliflower and the water to pan; bring to the boil. Reduce heat; cook, covered with a tight-fitting lid, about 15 minutes or until water is absorbed and quinoa is tender. Remove from heat, stir in kale; stand, covered, 10 minutes. Fluff with a fork. Stir in nuts and coriander.

3 Thread prawns onto 12 bamboo skewers. Cook skewers on a heated grill plate (or grill or barbecue) until prawns change colour.

4 Serve skewers with quinoa pilaf and lime wedges.

prep + cook time 45 minutes (+ refrigeration & standing)
serves 2
nutritional count per serving protein (48.6g), carbohydrate (57.7g), total fat (25.8g), fibre (16.5g).

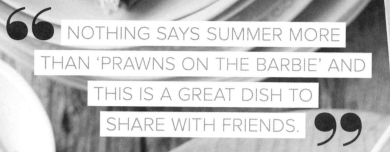

> NOTHING SAYS SUMMER MORE THAN 'PRAWNS ON THE BARBIE' AND THIS IS A GREAT DISH TO SHARE WITH FRIENDS.

cook's notes

You will need to soak 12 bamboo skewers in cold water for at least 30 minutes; this prevents skewers scorching during cooking.

cook's notes

You can use a cheaper cut of beef for this recipe, such as osso buco, gravy beef or chuck steak. If you don't want to use wine, you can add 2 tablespoons red wine vinegar instead. Similarly, you can substitute beef stock with 2 cups water and 1 tablespoon tamari.

beef ragu with zucchini pasta

2 tablespoons cold-pressed, extra-virgin, coconut oil

1kg (2 pounds) beef cheeks

1 small red onion (100g), chopped finely

1 large carrot (180g), chopped finely

2 stalks celery (300g), trimmed, chopped finely

1 small red capsicum (bell pepper) (150g), chopped finely

2 bay leaves

4 cloves garlic, crushed

2 drained anchovy fillets, chopped finely

¼ cup (70g) tomato paste

3 sprigs fresh thyme

3 sprigs fresh rosemary

½ cup (125ml) dry red wine

2 cups (500ml) beef stock

4 large zucchini (600g)

1 Preheat oven to 170°C/330°F.

2 Heat half the oil in a large flameproof casserole; season beef, cook, in batches, until browned. Remove from dish.

3 Heat the remaining oil in the dish; cook onion, carrot, celery, capsicum and bay leaves; stirring, over medium-low heat, about 5 minutes or until softened. Add garlic and anchovies; cook, stirring, 1 minute. Add tomato paste; cook, stirring, 1 minute.

4 Return beef to the dish; stir in the herbs, wine and stock. Bring to the boil. Cover dish.

5 Transfer dish to oven; cook, covered, about 3½ hours or until beef is very tender and falling apart. Remove dish from oven; discard herbs and bay leaves. Shred beef using two forks; season to taste.

6 Meanwhile, using a mandoline or v-slicer with a julienne attachment, slice the zucchini into long thin noodles/spaghetti.

7 Divide zucchini between serving bowls; top with hot beef ragu. Serve sprinkled with microherbs and a little shaved parmesan cheese, if you like.

prep + cook time 4 hours
serves 4
nutritional count per serving protein (62.8g), carbohydrate (10.5g), total fat (18.8g), fibre (6.3g).

chilli, ginger and lemon grass grilled chicken with rainbow salad

2 x 150g (5-ounce) chicken breast fillets

2cm (¾-inch) piece fresh ginger (10g), grated

10cm (4-inch) stick fresh lemon grass (20g), chopped very finely

½ fresh small red thai (serrano) chilli, chopped finely

1 tablespoon tamari

½ cup (100g) black rice

1½ cups (375ml) filtered water

1 cup (250ml) coconut milk

1 tablespoon cold-pressed extra-virgin coconut oil

1 lemon (140g), cut into wedges

RAINBOW SALAD

1 tablespoon tamari

1 tablespoon lemon juice

1 teaspoon roasted sesame oil

1 medium red capsicum (bell pepper) (200g), sliced thinly

75g (2½ ounces) snow peas, trimmed, sliced thinly lengthways

1 medium carrot (120g), cut into thin matchsticks

1 cup (80g) bean sprouts

1 cup loosely packed fresh mint leaves

1 Combine chicken, ginger, lemon grass, chilli and tamari in a medium bowl; toss well to combine. Cover; refrigerate 1 hour.

2 Meanwhile, place rice in a sieve; rinse under cold water until water runs clear. Combine the rice, the water and coconut milk in a medium saucepan; bring to the boil. Reduce heat to low, cover tightly; simmer, stirring occasionally, about 40 minutes or until rice is just tender and liquid is almost absorbed. Season to taste. Remove from heat; stand 10 minutes.

3 Stir oil into chicken mixture; cook chicken on a heated grill plate (or grill or barbecue), about 3 minutes each side or until cooked through. Remove chicken from heat; cover; stand 10 minutes.

4 Meanwhile, to make the rainbow salad, whisk tamari, juice and oil in a medium bowl until combined. Add the remaining ingredients; toss gently.

5 Serve chicken with rice, salad and lemon wedges.

prep + cook time 1 hour 30 minutes
serves 2
nutritional count per serving protein (47.3g), carbohydrate (53.1g), total fat (46.1g), fibre (11.3g).

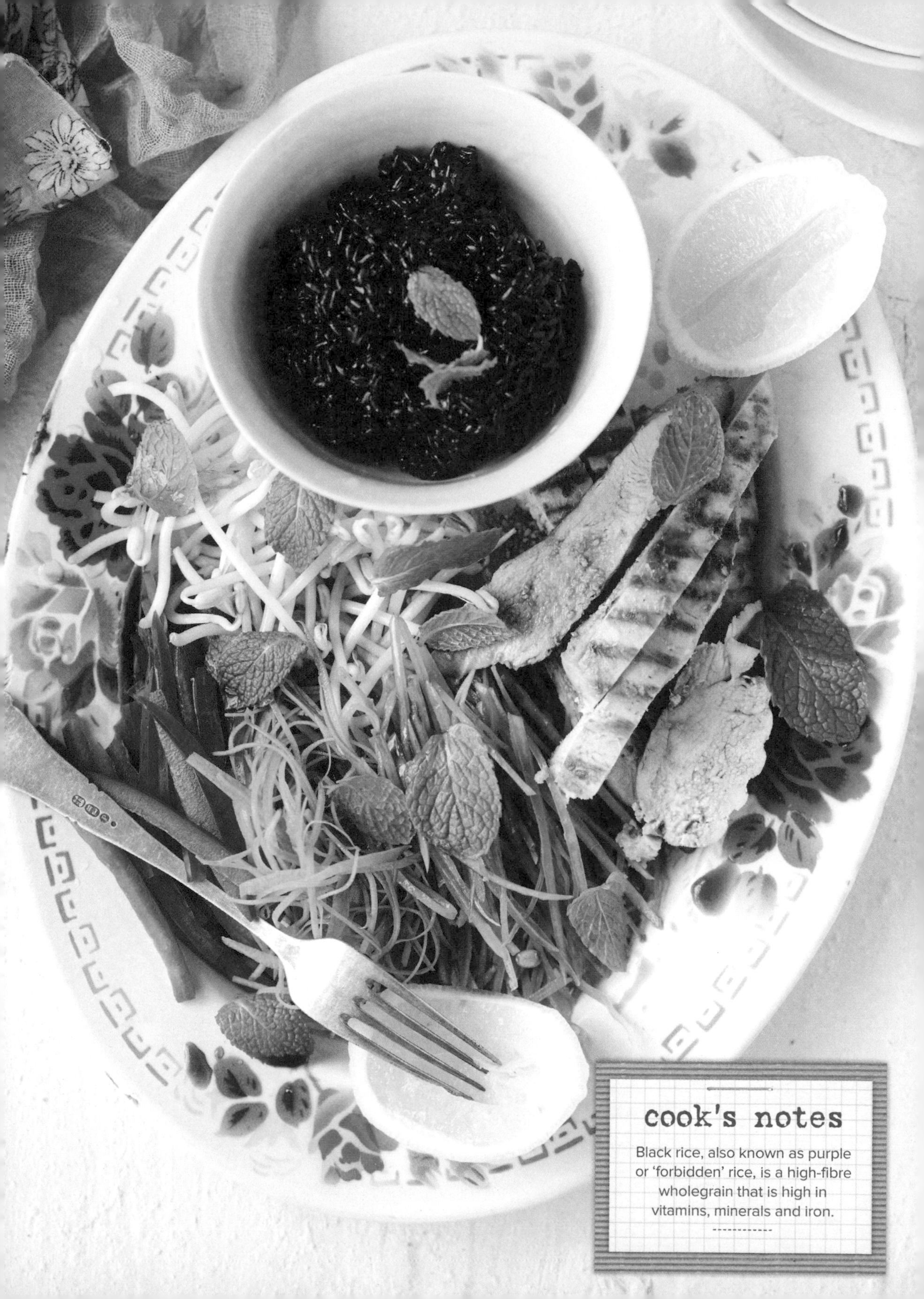

cook's notes

Black rice, also known as purple or 'forbidden' rice, is a high-fibre wholegrain that is high in vitamins, minerals and iron.

CHILLI AND GARLIC PRAWN
SKEWERS WITH QUINOA AND
CAULIFLOWER PILAF PAGE 168.

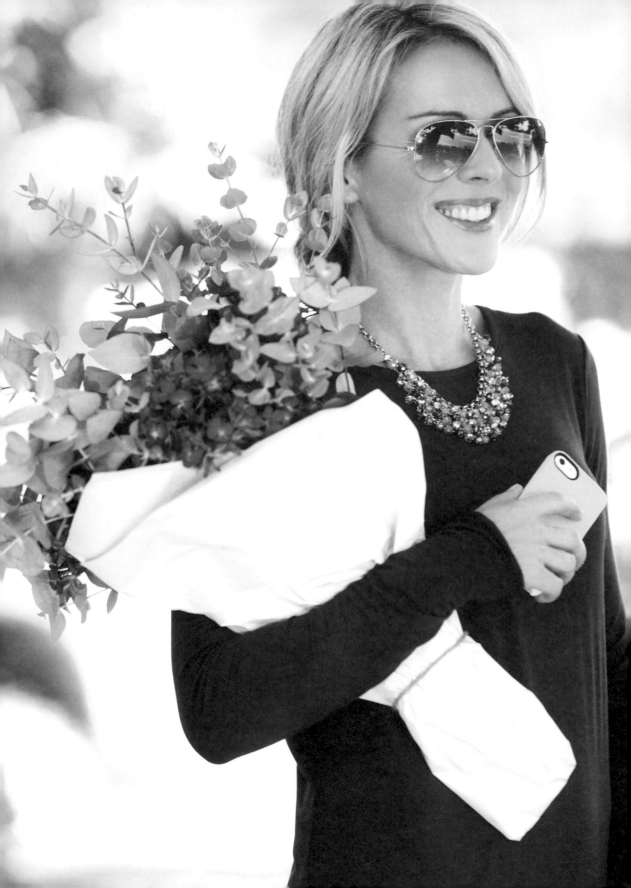

SEAFOOD PAELLA

1 tablespoon cold-pressed
extra-virgin coconut oil

1 small red onion (100g), chopped finely

3 cloves garlic, crushed

2 stalks celery (300g), trimmed, diced

1 medium red capsicum (bell pepper)
(200g), diced

1 teaspoon each ground fennel, ground
cumin and paprika

2 tablespoons tomato paste

1 cup (200g) brown short-grain rice

pinch saffron threads

1 bay leaf

3 medium tomatoes (450g),
chopped coarsely

2½ cups (625ml) filtered water

1 tablespoon tamari

75g (2½ ounces) green beans, trimmed,
chopped coarsely

1 cup (30g) baby spinach leaves

300g (9½ ounces) firm white fish fillets, cut
into 5cm (2-inch) pieces

6 uncooked medium king prawns (shrimp)
(270g), shelled, deveined, tails intact

6 scallops, roe removed (150g)

¼ cup loosely packed
fresh flat-leaf parsley leaves

1 lemon (140g), cut into wedges

1 Heat oil in a medium deep frying pan.
Cook onion and garlic, stirring, until onion
softens. Add celery, capsicum, fennel, cumin,
paprika and tomato paste; cook, stirring,
2 minutes or until vegetables are tender. Add
rice, saffron and bay leaf; stir to coat rice in
vegetable mixture.

2 Add tomatoes and ½ cup of the water;
cook, stirring, until liquid is absorbed. Add
remaining water and tamari; cook, covered,
over medium-low heat, stirring occasionally,
about 45 minutes or until liquid is absorbed
and rice is tender.

3 Stir beans and spinach into rice mixture.
Top with fish, prawns and scallops. Cook,
covered, about 5 minutes or until seafood is
just cooked through. Season to taste.

4 Cover paella; stand 5 minutes. Sprinkle
paella with parsley; serve with lemon
wedges.

prep + cook time 1 hour 40 minutes
serves 2
nutritional count per serving protein (73g),
carbohydrate (93.8g), total fat (16g), fibre (12.1g).

cook's notes

For a vegetarian option, omit the seafood and add 300g (9½ ounces) chopped mixed mushrooms with the capsicum in step 1.

We used bream fillets for this recipe but you can use any firm white fish fillets you like.

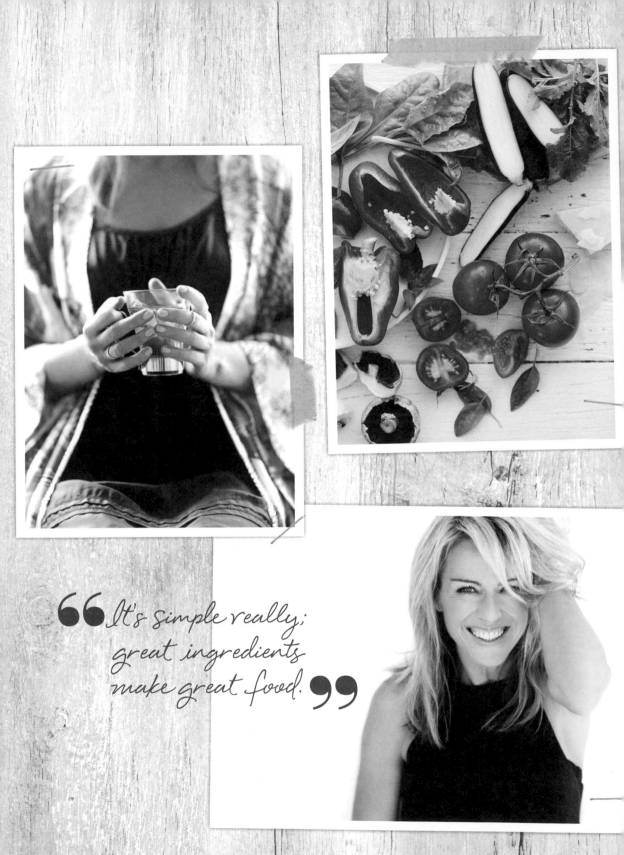

It's simple really;
great ingredients
make great food.

VEGETARIAN LASAGNE WITH
SHAVED FENNEL SALAD PAGE 180

vegetarian lasagne with shaved fennel salad

2 large red capsicums (bell peppers) (700g)

3 flat mushrooms (240g)

2 medium eggplants (600g)

2 medium kumara
(orange sweet potato) (800g)

3 large zucchinis (450g)

1 tablespoon cold-pressed
extra-virgin coconut oil

1½ cups (40g) baby spinach leaves

½ cup loosely packed fresh basil leaves

cook's notes

The lasagne makes enough for
6 serves. Freeze leftover slices
of lasagne, in individual airtight
containers, for up to 3 months.
Defrost lasagne slices overnight
in the fridge, then reheat in
a 180°C/350°F oven for
10-15 minutes.

TOMATO SAUCE

1 teaspoon cold-pressed
extra-virgin coconut oil

1 small brown onion (80g), chopped finely

2 cloves garlic, crushed

5 medium ripe tomatoes (750g),
chopped coarsely

WHITE SAUCE

2 tablespoons cold-pressed
extra-virgin coconut oil

2 tablespoons coconut flour

1 cup (250ml) almond mylk

1 teaspoon paprika

1 cup (80g) grated parmesan
or pecorino cheese

SHAVED FENNEL SALAD

2 medium fennel (600g)

1 small red onion (100g), sliced finely

4 cups (120g) baby rocket (arugula) leaves

¼ cup (60ml) lemon juice

1 Preheat oven to 200°C/400°F.

2 Quarter capsicums; discard seeds and membranes. Cut each piece into 3 thick strips. Slice mushrooms thinly. Cut eggplants, kumara and zucchinis lengthways into thin slices. Place half the vegetables, in single layer, on two baking-paper-lined oven trays; drizzle with the oil, season. Roast about 15 minutes or until browned and tender. Repeat with remaining vegetables. Place warm capsicum in a snaplock bag; stand 5 minutes. When cool enough to handle, peel away skins.

3 Meanwhile, to make the tomato sauce, heat oil in a medium saucepan; cook onion and garlic, stirring, until onion softens. Add tomatoes; simmer, covered, about 15 minutes or until sauce is thick. Season to taste.

4 To make the white sauce, heat oil in a small saucepan; add flour, cook, stirring, 2 minutes. Gradually add milk; cook, stirring, until mixture boils and thickens. Remove from heat; stir in paprika and half the cheese. Season to taste.

5 Cover the base of an 8 cup (2-litre) ovenproof dish with a layer of roasted vegetables, spinach and basil, overlapping slightly so there are no gaps. Top with half the tomato sauce.

6 Repeat another layer of vegetables. Top with remaining tomato sauce. Top with remaining basil and spinach. Carefully pour the white sauce over the top; sprinkle with the remaining cheese. Bake lasagne about 20 minutes or until golden brown and heated through.

7 Meanwhile, to make the fennel salad; trim fennel, reserve 1 tablespoon coarsely chopped fennel fronds. Using a mandoline or v-slicer, slice fennel and onion finely. Combine fennel, onion and reserved fronds in a medium bowl with the rocket and juice; toss gently. Season to taste.

8 Stand lasagne 5 minutes before serving with fennel salad.

----

prep + cook time 1 hour 45 minutes
serves 6
nutritional count per serving (with fennel salad) protein (17.1g), carbohydrate (34.9g), total fat (20.7g), fibre (13.3g).

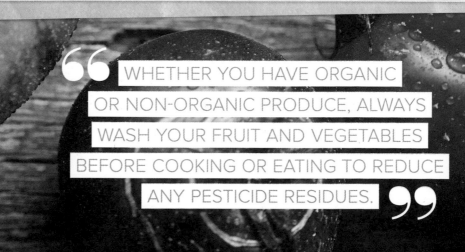

WHETHER YOU HAVE ORGANIC OR NON-ORGANIC PRODUCE, ALWAYS WASH YOUR FRUIT AND VEGETABLES BEFORE COOKING OR EATING TO REDUCE ANY PESTICIDE RESIDUES.

We used snapper for this recipe but you can use any firm white fish fillets you like.

SPICED FISH WITH QUINOA TABOULEH AND EGGPLANT PUREE

1 large eggplant (500g)

½ teaspoon each ground cumin, ground coriander and paprika

2 x 200g (6½-ounce) firm white fish fillets

2 teaspoons lemon juice

1 clove garlic, quartered

1 lemon (140g), cut into wedges

QUINOA TABOULEH

¾ cup (150g) dried white quinoa

1 cup (250ml) filtered water

2 tablespoons lemon juice

1 medium tomato (150g), chopped finely

1 lebanese cucumber (130g), seeded, chopped finely

½ cup each loosely packed fresh flat-leaf parsley and mint leaves

2 green onions (scallions), chopped finely

1 Preheat oven to 200°C/400°F.

2 Trim top from eggplant. Place eggplant on an oven tray; pierce all over with a fork. Roast about 30 minutes or until beginning to collapse. Remove from oven; cool.

3 Meanwhile, to make the quinoa tabouleh, rinse quinoa well; drain. Place quinoa in a small saucepan with the water; bring to the boil. Reduce heat; cook quinoa, covered with a tight-fitting lid, about 15 minutes or until water is absorbed and quinoa is tender. Remove from heat; stand, covered, 10 minutes. Fluff with a fork. Stir in the remaining ingredients. Season to taste.

4 Rub combined spices all over fish, season; place on oven tray. Roast about 10 minutes or until cooked as desired.

5 Peel eggplant; chop flesh coarsely. Process eggplant with juice and garlic until smooth; season to taste.

6 Serve fish with quinoa tabouleh, eggplant puree and lemon wedges.

prep + cook time 45 minutes
serves 2
nutritional count per serving protein (55.2g), carbohydrate (58.8g), total fat (8.8g), fibre (14.7g).

fennel and orange baked fish with roasted carrot and parsnip salad

1 baby fennel (130g)

400g (12½ ounces) baby carrots, trimmed, peeled

2 medium parsnips (500g), quartered

1 small red onion (100g), cut into wedges

¼ cup (60ml) orange juice

1½ tablespoons cold-pressed extra-virgin coconut oil

2 teaspoons finely grated orange rind

1 teaspoon fennel seeds

2 x 200g (6½-ounce) firm white fish fillets

1 tablespoon macadamia oil

1 tablespoon apple cider vinegar

2 cups baby rocket (arugula) leaves

1 lemon, cut into wedges

1 Preheat oven to 200°C/400°F.

2 Trim fennel; reserve 1 tablespoon finely chopped fennel fronds. Cut fennel into thin wedges.

3 Combine fennel, carrots, parsnip, onion, 2 tablespoons of the orange juice and 1 tablespoon of the coconut oil in a medium baking dish; roast 20 minutes.

4 Rub combined remaining coconut oil, rind and fennel seeds all over fish, season. Remove dish from oven; place fish on top of vegetables. Roast about 10 minutes or until fish is cooked as desired and vegetables are browned and tender.

5 Meanwhile, whisk oil, vinegar, reserved fennel fronds and the remaining orange juice in a medium bowl until combined.

6 Remove dish from oven; transfer fish to plate, cover to keep warm. Add vegetables and rocket to bowl with dressing; toss gently.

7 Serve fish with salad, lemon wedges and extra fennel fronds, if you like.

prep + cook time 45 minutes
serves 2
nutritional count per serving
protein (48.8g), carbohydrate (37.2g), total fat (27.3g), fibre (17.1g)

We used blue-eye cod for this recipe but you can use any firm white fish you like.

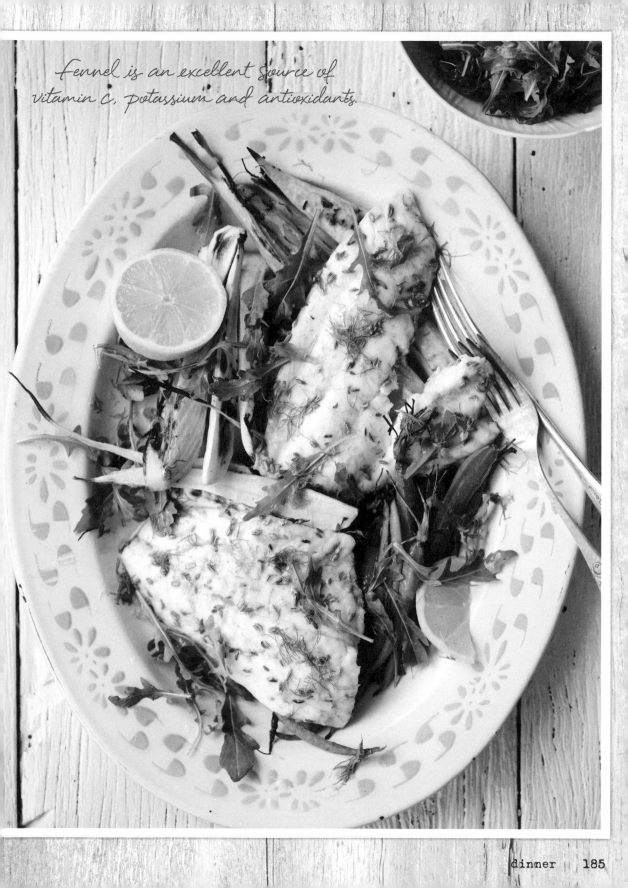

Fennel is an excellent source of vitamin c, potassium and antioxidants.

"DON'T CHANGE
SO PEOPLE WILL LIKE YOU

BE
YOURSELF

AND THE RIGHT PEOPLE WILL

LOVE THE
REAL YOU."

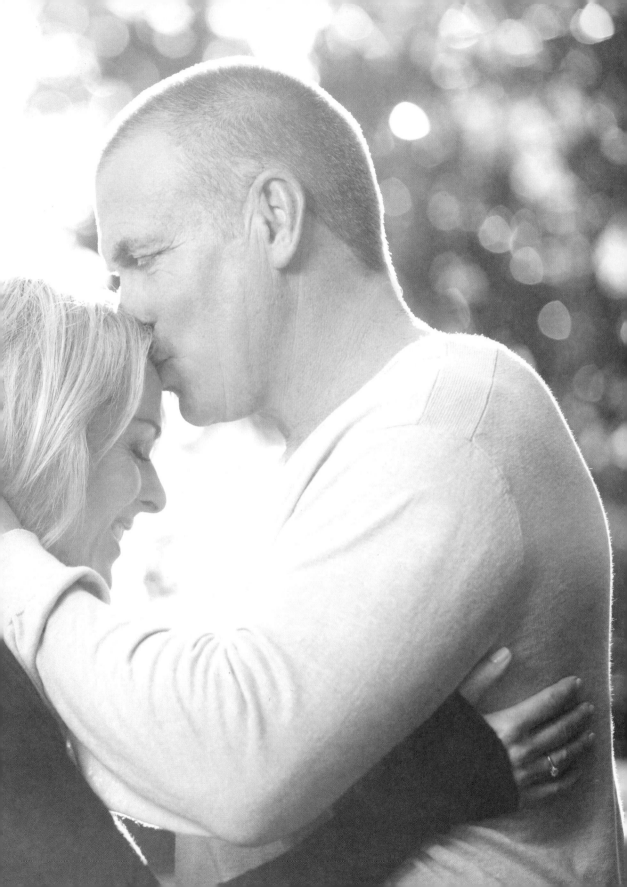

tamari, lime and sesame beef and broccoli stir-fry

2 tablespoons cold-pressed extra-virgin coconut oil

300g (9½ ounces) beef eye-fillet, sliced thinly

1 clove garlic, crushed

2cm (¾-inch) piece fresh ginger (10g), grated

½ fresh long red chilli, sliced thinly

100g (3 ounces) fresh shiitake mushrooms, sliced thickly

400g (12 ½ ounces) gai lan (chinese broccoli), leaves separated, stems chopped coarsely

300g (9½ ounces) broccoli, halved, sliced thickly

115g (3½ ounces) baby corn, halved lengthways

¼ cup (60ml) filtered water

¾ cup (180ml) vegetable stock

2 tablespoons tamari

1 tablespoon lime juice

1 teaspoon sesame oil

½ teaspoon each of toasted black and white sesame seeds

¼ cup loosely packed fresh thai basil leaves

1 lime, cut into wedges

1 Heat half the coconut oil in a wok. Combine beef with garlic and ginger in small bowl; stir-fry in wok, in batches, until browned. Remove from wok.
2 Heat remaining coconut oil in wok; stir fry chilli, mushrooms, gai lan stems, broccoli and corn with the water, until vegetables are tender.
3 Add gai lan leaves, stock, tamari, juice and sesame oil; stir-fry until hot. Season to taste.
4 Sprinkle with seeds and thai basil leaves; serve with lime wedges.

prep + cook time 35 minutes
serves 2
nutritional count per serving protein (55.6g), carbohydrate (15.2g), total fat (31.1g), fibre (18.7g).

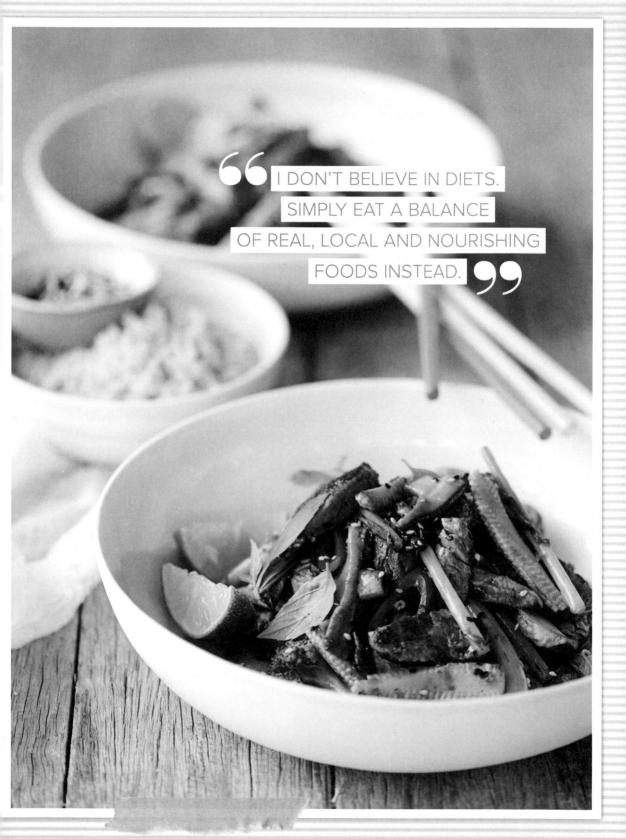

"I DON'T BELIEVE IN DIETS. SIMPLY EAT A BALANCE OF REAL, LOCAL AND NOURISHING FOODS INSTEAD."

cook's notes

We used barramundi for this recipe but you can use any firm white fish fillets you like.

If chinese vegetables are unavailable, you can use broccolini, asparagus or kale.

----

chilli, honey and tamari fish bundles with asian greens

1 fresh long red chilli

500g (1 pound) gai lan (chinese broccoli), trimmed, cut into 5cm (2-inch) lengths

500g (1 pound) baby buk choy, halved

75g (2½ ounces) snow peas, trimmed

2 x 200g (6½-ounces) firm white fish fillets

2 tablespoons tamari

2 tablespoons cold-pressed extra-virgin coconut oil

1 clove garlic, crushed

1cm (½-inch) piece fresh ginger (5g), grated

2 teaspoons raw honey

1 tablespoon finely chopped fresh coriander leaves

⅓ cup loosely packed fresh coriander (cilantro) leaves

1 lime, cut into wedges

1 Preheat oven to 200°C/400°F.

2 Finely chop half the chilli; thinly slice remaining chilli.

3 Place two 30cm (12-inch) squares baking paper on a board. Divide gai lan, buk choy and snow peas between squares of paper. Place fish on top of vegetables.

4 Whisk tamari, oil, garlic, ginger, honey, chopped coriander and chopped chilli in a small bowl until combined. Drizzle tamari mixture over fish. Gather corners of baking paper together above fish; twist to enclose securely.

5 Place parcels on oven tray; bake about 15 minutes or until cooked as desired.

6 Serve bundles open on serving plates; sprinkle with sliced chilli and coriander leaves. Serve with lime wedges.

prep + cook time 35 minutes
serves 2
nutritional count per serving protein (59.8g), carbohydrate (13.5g), total fat (23g), fibre (15.7g).

Serve with coconut rice or steamed black rice, if you like.

roasted pumpkin, beetroot, chickpea and barley salad

½ cup (100g) dried chickpeas
(garbanzo beans)

½ cup (100g) pearl barley

150g (4½ ounces) green beans, trimmed

500g (1 pound) pumpkin, unpeeled,
sliced thinly

4 baby beetroot (beets) (100g), peeled,
trimmed, quartered or halved

50g (1½ ounces) soft goat's cheese, crumbled

2 tablespoons toasted pepitas
(pumpkin seeds)

MAPLE AND THYME DRESSING

2 tablespoons cold-pressed
extra-virgin olive oil

2 tablespoons pure maple syrup

2 tablespoons white wine vinegar

2 teaspoons fresh thyme leaves

1 Place chickpeas in a small bowl, cover with cold water; stand overnight, drain.

2 Preheat oven to 200°C/400°F.

3 Cook chickpeas and barley in a medium saucepan of boiling filtered water, about 20 minutes or until tender. Add green beans to pan in last 1 minute of cooking time; drain. Rinse under cold water; drain.

4 Meanwhile, to make the maple and thyme dressing, combine ingredients in a screw-top jar, season to taste; shake well to combine.

5 Combine pumpkin and beetroot with 2 tablespoons of the dressing in a small baking-paper-lined baking dish. Roast about 20 minutes or until caramelised and tender.

6 Combine barley, chickpeas, beans, pumpkin and beetroot with spinach and remaining dressing in a medium bowl; toss gently. Serve salad sprinkled with cheese and pepitas.

prep + cook time 35 minutes (+ standing)
serves 2
nutritional count per serving protein (35g), carbohydrate (75.1g), total fat (42.2g), fibre (24.1g).

This is one of my fave 'meatless Monday' dishes, but it is equally delicious with some poached chicken shredded on top.

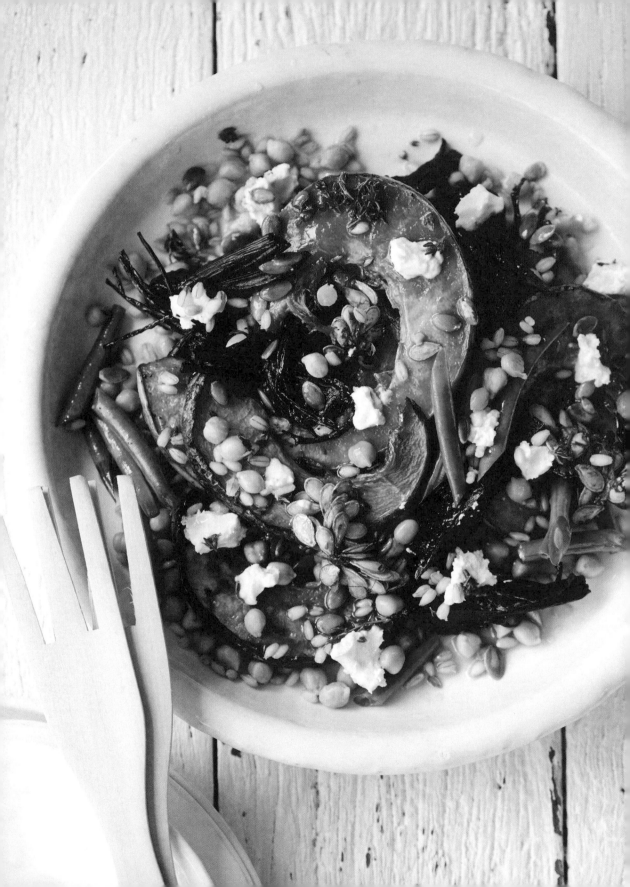

Salmon is high in protein, rich in anti-inflammatory omega 3 and a good source of vitamin b.

GRILLED MISO SALMON WITH BEAN AND PEA SALAD

1 tablespoon white (shiro) miso paste

1 tablespoon tamari

2cm (¾-inch) piece fresh ginger (10g), grated

1 teaspoon finely grated lemon rind

1 teaspoon sesame oil

2 x 200g (6½-ounce) boneless salmon fillets, skin on

175g (5½ ounces) asparagus, trimmed

75g (2½ ounces) green beans, trimmed

75g (2½ ounces) snow peas, trimmed

75g (2½ ounces) sugar snap peas, trimmed

1 cup (120g) frozen peas

1 lemon (140g), cut into wedges

⅓ cup loosely packed fresh coriander (cilantro) leaves

2 green onions (scallions), cut into fine strips

1 tablespoon toasted sesame seeds

LEMON SESAME DRESSING

2 tablespoons lemon juice

1 teaspoon sesame oil

1 Combine miso, tamari, ginger, rind and oil in a medium bowl; add salmon, toss to coat in mixture.

2 Steam asparagus, beans, snow peas, sugar snap peas and peas, over a medium saucepan of boiling water, until just tender. Drain. Rinse under cold water; drain.

3 Meanwhile, cook salmon in a heated grill pan (or grill or barbecue) about 3 minutes each side or until cooked as desired. Cover; stand 5 minutes.

4 To make lemon sesame dressing, whisk the ingredients in a medium bowl until combined. Add asparagus, beans and all the peas; mix well. Season to taste.

5 Serve salmon with bean mixture and lemon wedges; sprinkle with coriander, onion and sesame seeds.

prep + cook time 35 minutes
serves 2
nutritional count per serving protein (70.2g), carbohydrate (13.8g), total fat (34.3g), fibre (11.8g).

mustard beef
with kumara mash

500g (1 pound) piece beef eye-fillet

1 tablespoon red wine vinegar

1 teaspoon wholegrain mustard

1 teaspoon fresh thyme leaves

1 clove garlic, crushed

2 teaspoons cold-pressed
extra-virgin coconut oil

2 tablespoons red wine vinegar, extra

½ teaspoon wholegrain mustard, extra

⅓ cup (80ml) beef stock

½ teaspoon arrowroot

2 teaspoons filtered water

KUMARA MASH

1 large kumara (orange sweet potato)
(500g), chopped coarsely

1 clove garlic, peeled

1 sprig fresh thyme

TOMATO AND MESCLUN SALAD

200g (6½ ounces) mixed baby
tomatoes, halved

30g (1 ounce) baby mesclun
salad leaves

2 teaspoons red wine vinegar

1 teaspoon cold-pressed
extra-virgin, coconut oil

1 Tie beef at 2cm (¾-inch) intervals with kitchen string. Combine vinegar, mustard, thyme and garlic in a medium bowl; add beef, toss to coat beef in mustard mixture. Cover; refrigerate 3 hours or overnight.

2 Preheat oven to 200°C/400°F.

3 Add coconut oil to beef. Heat a small flameproof baking dish; cook beef, turning, until browned all over.

4 Transfer dish to oven; roast beef, about 20 minutes or until cooked as desired.

5 Meanwhile, to make the kumara mash, steam kumara with garlic and thyme over a medium pan of boiling water, about 15 minutes, or until tender. Drain. Discard thyme and garlic; mash kumara in a small bowl until smooth.

6 Remove beef from dish; wrap in aluminium foil. Stand 10 minutes.

7 Return dish with any pan juices to stove over low heat; add the extra vinegar, stirring. Add the extra mustard and stock. Dissolve arrowroot in the water in a small cup, add to dish. Cook, stirring, until sauce boils and thickens.

8 To make tomato and mesclun salad, combine ingredients in a medium bowl; toss gently. Season to taste.

9 Serve thickly sliced beef with mustard sauce, kumara mash and tomato and mesclun salad.

prep + cook time 1 hour (+ refrigeration)
serves 2
nutritional count per serving protein (57.9g), carbohydrate (32.2g), total fat (20g), fibre (5.9g).

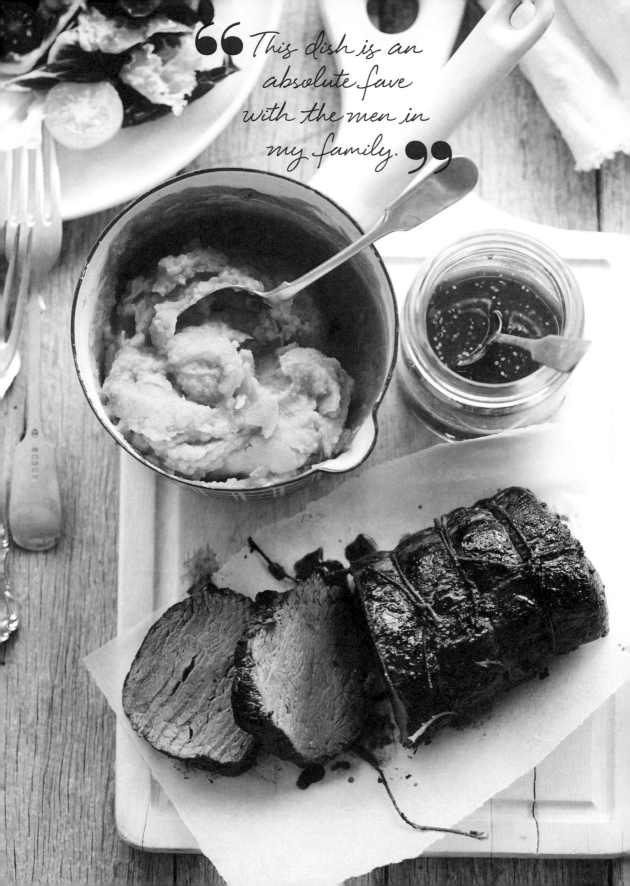

This dish is an absolute fave with the men in my family.

EATING OUT MADE EASY

eating out can be a minefield when it comes to staying on track with your health and wellbeing. And although I love to be social and try new things and new foods, eating out is not something I do on a regular basis.

YOU KNOW, I'LL BE THE FIRST TO SAY THAT YOU SHOULD ENJOY FOOD WITHOUT ANY FEELINGS OF GUILT, AND I OFTEN GO TO AMAZING RESTAURANTS AND EAT EXACTLY WHAT I FEEL LIKE (AND I ENCOURAGE YOU TO DO THE SAME). BUT I HAVE TO STRESS THAT IT'S REALLY IMPORTANT THAT YOU ONLY DO IT ONCE OR TWICE A WEEK AND DEFINITELY NOT ALL THE TIME.

When eating out, the first thing you need to consider is the quality of the place where you have chosen to dine. I try to choose places that value fresh produce, have ethical standards when it comes to their meats and produce and have a great reputation for taste and nutrition. This is important to me because I don't believe I should disregard my beliefs or lower my standards when it comes to my nutrition just because the food is not coming from my own kitchen.

That being said, when I'm travelling or having to eat out a little more than I would like, I use the following guidelines to help me stay on track:

HERE ARE A FEW THINGS I DO TO STAY ON TRACK

* I skip the starter and just order a main course. If I am really hungry I will order a salad, fresh juice or ginger tea (if it's on the menu).

* I choose meals that I can add healthy sides to, like fish, or a grass-fed steak. Then I look at how it is cooked, always asking for it to be grilled or steamed, knowing it will have the same delicious flavour, but be healthier for me.

* If it comes with a sauce, I ask for the sauce on the side, just adding a tiny bit at a time to get the same great taste that the chef intended.

* When choosing sides I opt for green foods such as brussels sprouts, broccoli, spinach (not creamed), salads and beans and avoid things like creamy mashed potato and fries.

* If I'm having Italian, I choose tomato-based sauces over the cheese or cream ones, and go easy on the parmesan. Likewise, if I'm eating Asian food, I look for stir-fried vegetable-based dishes and avoid the sauces that are laden with salt, cream or fats.

* If I feel like dessert, I try to choose the lightest option, which might be a sorbet, or a fruit-based dish. If there is something on the menu I simply can't resist I ask someone to share it with me. I find it is the first couple of spoonfuls that taste the best and that is usually the perfect amount to satisfy my cravings and my curiosity.

* I like to finish my meal with a soothing herbal tea, and most restaurants now have at least peppermint (one of my favourites) or chamomile on the menu.

I THINK THE MOST IMPORTANT THINGS TO REMEMBER WHEN EATING OUT ARE THAT YOU SHOULD MAKE THE HEALTHIEST CHOICES POSSIBLE WITH WHAT IS AVAILABLE, RELAX AND ENJOY YOUR TIME WITH FAMILY AND FRIENDS AND THEN GET RIGHT BACK TO YOUR HEALTHY EATING THE VERY NEXT DAY.

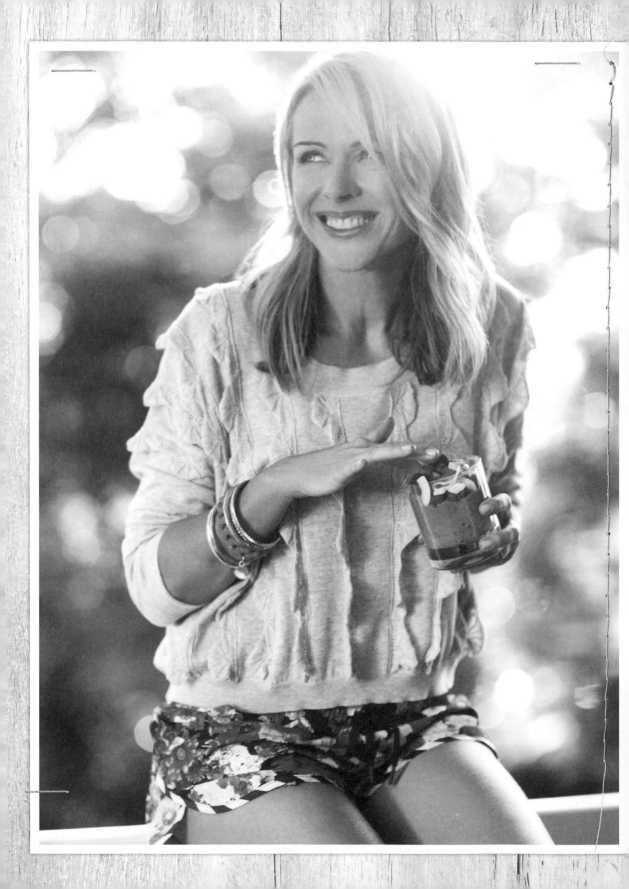

DESSERTS

I've always had a sweet tooth and more often than not find myself reaching for something sweet after dinner. Now I'm not saying you should treat yourself to a dessert every night, but if you're going to eat something sweet, it's incredibly important that you make sure it's as nutrient rich and delicious as humanly possible.

I treat dessert as my third snack for the day and leave a little time between having it and finishing dinner. That way I don't overload my digestive system just before going to bed and it also gives me a little time to decide whether I really want it.

The desserts I have chosen for this book are nothing short of spectacular. Many are based on fruit, none are excessively sweet and all are served in moderate portions.

I promise you - they will taste so good that you won't believe they are actually good for you!

REFRESH WATERMELON 'CAKE'

1kg (2-pound) large round piece of seedless watermelon

1 lime

2 teaspoons raw honey

2 cups (480g) ricotta cheese

3 medium fresh figs (120g), quartered or halved

2 tablespoons coarsely chopped roasted unsalted shelled pistachios

¼ cup loosely packed fresh small mint leaves

2 teaspoons raw honey, extra

1 Remove skin and rind from watermelon, keeping the flesh as a whole round piece.
2 Using a vegetable peeler, peel rind thinly from the lime. Cut lime rind into long, fine strips. Juice lime; reserve 2 tablespoons juice.
3 Combine lime juice and honey in a small bowl; stir in ricotta.
4 Place watermelon piece on serving plate; spread ricotta mixture on top. Pile figs on top; sprinkle with nuts, mint and lime rind.
5 Drizzle with extra honey before serving, cut into wedges.

prep time 20 minutes
serves 8
nutritional count per serving protein (7g), carbohydrate (11.8g), total fat (7.8g), fibre (1.7g).

Sometimes I cover the sides of the watermelon slice with ricotta as well for maximum impact when I slice it at the table.

cook's notes

Labne, or labneh, is a soft cream cheese made from strained yoghurt. It is low in kilojoules so is a good substitute for cream. You need to make the vanilla labne 24 hours ahead of time, for this recipe.

----

pear and berry crumbles with vanilla labne

2 medium pears (460g), peeled, cored, cut into 1.5cm (¾-inch) pieces

1 teaspoon raw honey

2 tablespoons filtered water

1½ (185g) cups fresh or frozen mixed berries

⅓ cup (55g) almond kernels, chopped coarsely

⅓ cup (45g) macadamias, chopped coarsely

⅓ cup (50g) brown rice flour

1 teaspoon ground cinnamon

2 tablespoons rolled oats

1 tablespoon pepitas (pumpkin seeds)

1 tablespoon white chia seeds

2 tablespoons cold-pressed extra-virgin coconut oil

1 tablespoon raw honey, extra

VANILLA LABNE

1 cup (280g) unsweetened greek yoghurt

pinch Himalayan pink salt

1 teaspoon vanilla bean paste

1 To make vanilla labne, combine yoghurt and salt in a small bowl. Line a sieve with two layers of muslin or a clean cloth; place sieve over a deep bowl or jug. Spoon yoghurt mixture into sieve, gather cloth and tie into a ball with kitchen string. Refrigerate overnight, or until the mixture thickens, gently squeezing occasionally to encourage the liquid to drain. Discard liquid. Stir vanilla into labne.

2 Preheat oven to 170°C/350°F.

3 Combine pear, honey and the water in a small saucepan; bring to the boil. Reduce heat; simmer, covered, about 5 minutes or until pear is just tender. Remove from heat; stir in berries. Divide pear mixture into 2 x 1½ cup (375ml) ovenproof dishes or jars.

4 Combine nuts, flour, cinnamon, oats, pepitas and chia seeds in a medium bowl. Add coconut oil and extra honey; mix well. Spoon crumble mixture over fruit (piling crumble high on top of fruit as it will sink down a little during cooking).

5 Bake crumbles about 20 minutes or until crumble topping is golden and crisp. Serve with vanilla labne.

prep + cook time 40 minutes (+ refrigeration)
serves 2
nutritional count per serving protein (24.3g), carbohydrate (91.4g), total fat (63g), fibre (7.1g).

THE LOW-DOWN ON SUGAR AND SWEETENERS

DID YOU KNOW THAT SUGAR IS MORE ADDICTIVE THAN COCAINE?

It is not a nutrient. It causes wrinkles and bad skin, suppresses your immune system, causes diabetes, kidney and heart problems and is bad for your teeth and overall good health.

Over the years, we have been ill-advised in our quest for sweetness and there have been numerous artificial sweeteners included in our 'health foods'. But beware – the reality is that artificial 'anything' is bad for your health and some artificial sweeteners have even been linked to chronic disease and even terminal illnesses like cancer.

MY BELIEF IS THAT NATURAL IS ALWAYS BETTER AND THERE'S A WIDE VARIETY OF NUTRITIOUS AND DELICIOUS NATURAL SWEETENERS READILY AVAILABLE FOR YOU TO USE.

Some of my favourite sweeteners are:

DATES

I use them regularly in baking
and for my smoothies.

RAW ORGANIC HONEY

One of the oldest unrefined sweeteners that I use to
sweeten my oats and tonics and tea.

MAPLE SYRUP

Contains a wide range of minerals and antioxidants that are great for
your health and because of its distinct taste you only need a little to
add delicious sweetness to your food.

COCONUT NECTAR

I use it in tonics and for baking.

RAPADURA SUGAR

Great for baking.

STEVIA LEAVES

I grow this in my garden and grind it myself because I've found that
when buying this in shops, it tends to be just as overly processed and
bleached as white sugar most of the time.

If you have a sweet tooth, I would recommend trying delicious
fresh fruits to add sweetness to your diet or one of these less processed
sugar alternatives that are still as close to their natural state as possible.
But remember – you're sweet enough as it is, so use them in moderation
and ALWAYS buy them from your farmer's market or local produce
or health food store to guarantee their purity.

RHUBARB AND COCONUT CREAM CUPS

⅓ cup (15g) flaked coconut

2 tablespoons coarsely chopped unsalted shelled pistachios

2 tablespoons pepitas (pumpkin seeds)

2 tablespoons sunflower seed kernels

2 teaspoons white chia seeds

500g (1 pound) rhubarb, trimmed, cut into 2.5cm (1-inch) lengths

2 tablespoons pure maple syrup

2 teaspoons finely grated orange rind

⅓ cup (80ml) orange juice

1 vanilla bean, split lengthways

COCONUT AND CASHEW CREAM

½ cup (75g) unsalted cashews

1 cup (100g) young coconut flesh

2 teaspoons pure maple syrup

¼ cup (60ml) pure coconut water

1 To make the coconut and cashew cream, soak nuts in a small bowl of filtered water for 30 minutes. Drain nuts. In a high speed blender, blend nuts, coconut flesh, maple syrup and enough coconut water until mixture is smooth and creamy (the amount of coconut water needed will depend on how much flesh you get out of your coconut and how firm it is).

2 Meanwhile, preheat oven to 170°C/330°F.

3 Place coconut, nuts and seeds on an oven tray; roast about 3 minutes or until browned lightly. Cool.

4 Meanwhile, combine rhubarb, maple syrup, rind, juice and vanilla bean in a small saucepan; bring to the boil. Reduce heat; simmer, uncovered, about 3 minutes or until rhubarb is just tender. Cool. Discard vanilla bean.

5 Layer rhubarb mixture, coconut and cashew cream and nut mixture in 2 x 1½ cup (375ml) serving glasses or jars. Serve.

prep + cook time 20 minutes
(+ standing & cooling)
serves 2
nutritional count per serving protein (24.8g), carbohydrate (44.2g), total fat (52.7g), fibre (11.9g).

cook's notes

You will need 1 young drinking coconut for this recipe. We used both the pure coconut water and the soft jelly-like flesh (which we scooped out with a spoon).

I love the impact of layered desserts — and often just layer the cream with fresh fruit in season.

yoghurt pops

See following
pages for recipes

MIXED BERRY AND CHIA
YOGHURT POPS

PASSIONFRUIT AND
MANGO YOGHURT POPS

CHOCOLATE, BANANA AND
ALMOND YOGHURT POPS

**SO DELICIOUS – THEY WON'T
BELIEVE THAT THEY'RE
GOOD FOR THEM!**

YOGHURT POPS

passionfruit and mango yoghurt pops

½ small mango (150g), chopped coarsely

½ cup (140g) unsweetened greek yoghurt

½ cup (125ml) passionfruit pulp

1 Process mango until smooth.
2 Combine mango puree, yoghurt and passionfruit in a medium jug. Pour mixture evenly into 6 x ¼-cup (60ml) ice-block moulds. Push in sticks.
3 Freeze 3 hours or overnight until firm.

prep + cook time 10 minutes (+ freezing)
makes 6
nutritional count per pop protein (2g), carbohydrate (6.6g), total fat (1.5g), fibre (3.2g).

cook's notes

For a non-dairy version of these frozen yoghurt pops, you could use store-bought coconut yoghurt or try making your own; see page 60 for recipe]

----

chocolate, banana and almond yoghurt pops

1 cup (280g) unsweetened greek yoghurt

2 tablespoons natural almond butter

1 tablespoon pure maple syrup

2 tablespoons cacao powder

1 small banana (130g), sliced thinly

1 Combine half the yoghurt, almond butter and half the maple syrup in a small bowl.

2 Combine the remaining yoghurt with the remaining maple syrup and sifted cacao powder in another small bowl.

3 Using the tip of your fingers, carefully press banana slices on the insides of 6 x ¼-cup (60ml) ice-block moulds. Layer almond mixture and cacao mixture into moulds, alternating which mixture you start with. Push in sticks.

4 Freeze 3 hours or overnight until firm.

prep + cook time 15 minutes (+ freezing)
makes 6
nutritional count per pop protein (4.6g), carbohydrate (13.1g), total fat (6.7g), fibre (0.4g).

mixed berry and chia yoghurt pops

¾ cup (200g) unsweetened greek yoghurt

1 cup (150g) fresh or frozen mixed berries

1 tablespoon black chia seeds

1 Process yoghurt with half the berries until smooth. Transfer mixture to a medium jug; stir in chia seeds; fold in the remaining berries.

2 Pour mixture evenly into 6 x ¼-cup (60ml) ice-block moulds. Push in sticks.

3 Freeze 3 hours or overnight until firm.

prep time 10 minutes (+ freezing)
makes 6
nutritional count per pop protein (2.4g), carbohydrate (6.9g), total fat (3g), fibre (0.6g).

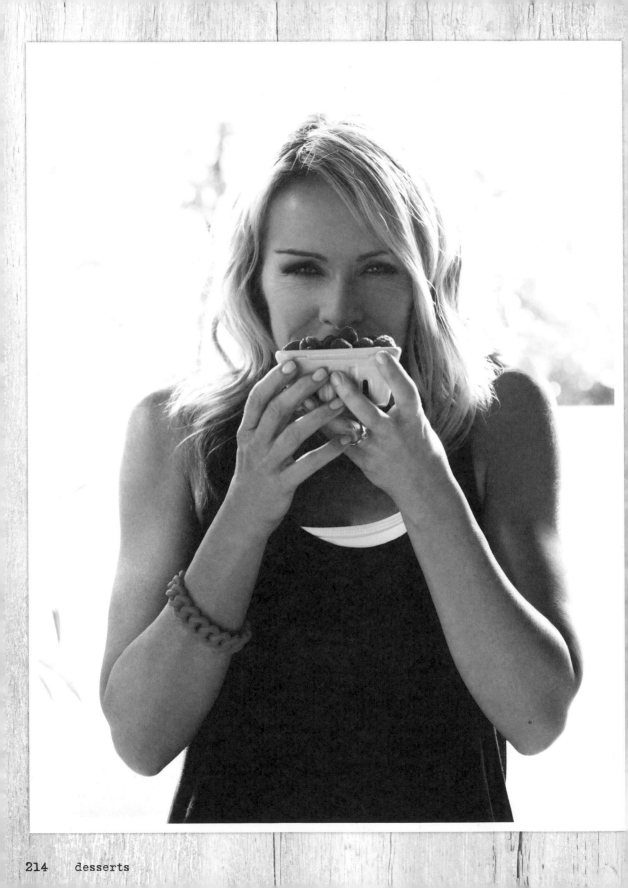

"NEVER REGRET ANYTHING, ESPECIALLY DESSERT."

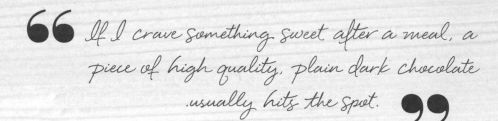
If I crave something sweet after a meal, a piece of high quality, plain dark chocolate usually hits the spot.

homemade raspberry and hazelnut chocolate

¼ cup (35g) coarsely chopped hazelnuts

⅓ cup (15g) flaked coconut

1 cup (110g) cacao butter, chopped finely

½ cup (50g) cacao powder

⅓ cup (80ml) raw honey or pure maple syrup

pinch Himalayan pink salt

½ cup (60g) fresh or frozen raspberries

1 Preheat oven to 170°C/330°F.

2 Place nuts and coconut on an oven tray; roast about 3 minutes or until browned lightly. Cool.

3 Meanwhile, place cacao butter in a medium heatproof bowl set over a medium saucepan of simmering water (do not let water touch base of bowl.) Stir cacao butter until it is melted. Remove from heat; stir in sifted cacao powder, honey (or maple syrup) and salt.

4 Pour cacao mixture onto a baking-paper-lined small oven tray. Sprinkle with nuts, coconut and berries. Freeze 30 minutes or until set. Break into pieces; store in freezer.

prep + cook time 20 minutes (+ freezing)
makes about 20 pieces
nutritional count per piece protein (1g), carbohydrate (5.7g), total fat (7.3g), fibre (0.4g).

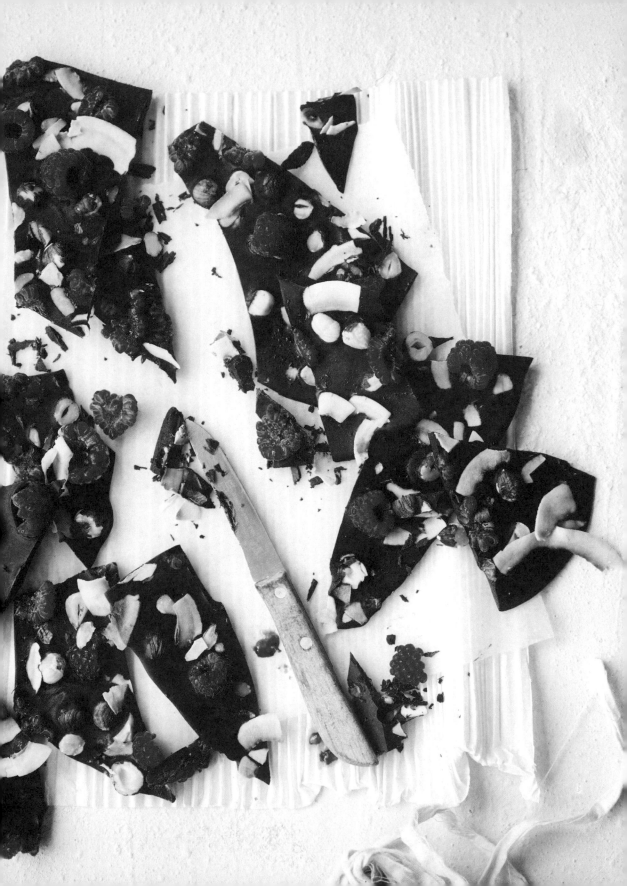

You will need to make
the ice-cream a day
ahead of serving.

BANANA, HONEY AND MACADAMIA ICE-CREAM SANDWICHES

1 cup (140g) macadamias

2 organic free-range egg yolks

2 tablespoons raw honey

pinch Himalayan pink salt

1¾ cups (400ml) coconut cream

½ cup mashed banana

MACADAMIA BISCUITS

1 cup (140g) macadamias

⅓ cup (75g) coconut sugar

1 teaspoon ground cinnamon

1 organic free-range egg white

1 Preheat oven to 180°C/350°F.

2 Place nuts on an oven tray; roast about 3 minutes or until browned lightly. Cool; chop nuts finely.

3 Whisk egg yolks and honey in a medium heatproof bowl set over a medium saucepan of simmering water; continue whisking for 5 minutes or until mixture is doubled in size and is white and fluffy.

4 Remove bowl from heat; whisk in salt, coconut cream and banana until well combined. Fold in the chopped nuts. Pour mixture into an ice-cream machine; following manufacturer's instructions, churn ice-cream for about 10 minutes or until the mixture has frozen considerably. Pour mixture into a loaf pan, cover with foil; freeze 4 hours or overnight. If you don't have an ice-cream machine, pour mixture into a loaf pan, cover with foil; freeze 4 hours, scraping sides of pan and mixing ice-cream well with a fork every 1 hour. Freeze overnight.

5 To make the macadamia biscuits, preheat oven to 170°C/330°F. Line two oven trays with baking paper.

6 Process nuts, sugar and cinnamon until fine. Transfer to a medium bowl; stir in egg white until mixture is combined. Drop level tablespoons of mixture onto trays, spread into 5cm circles. Bake about 12 minutes or until golden. Cool on trays.

7 Sandwich ice-cream between biscuits. Freeze until ready to serve.

prep + cook time 1 hour 30 minutes (+ freezing)
makes 6
nutritional count per ice-cream sandwich
protein (6.4g), carbohydrate (28.8g), total fat (50.5g), fibre (1g).

cook's notes

Biscuits can be made a day ahead; store in an airtight container. You can assemble the ice-cream sandwiches and keep them, between layers of baking paper, in an airtight container, in the freezer for up to 3 months.

oat and berry-stuffed baked peaches

½ cup (45g) rolled oats

⅓ cup (45g) dried cranberries

2 tablespoons dried blueberries

1 tablespoon shredded coconut

1 tablespoon pepitas (pumpkin seeds)

1 tablespoon raw honey

1 tablespoon cold-pressed extra-virgin coconut oil

2 large peaches (440g), halved, stones removed

greek yoghurt or coconut yoghurt, to serve

1 Preheat oven to 180°C/350°F.
2 Combine oats, berries, coconut, pepitas, honey and coconut oil in a small bowl.
3 Place peach halves, cut side up on an oven tray; firmly press oat mixture into cavities, piling mixture high.
4 Bake peaches about 20 minutes or until topping is golden and peaches are tender. Serve with greek-style yoghurt or coconut yoghurt, if you like.

prep + cook time 35 minutes
serves 2
nutritional count per serving protein (7.2g), carbohydrate (50.5g), total fat (18.4g), fibre (6.7g).

cook's notes

When peaches are not in season you can use apples instead. Core whole apples, making a 2.5cm (1-inch) wide cavity, without cutting all the way through the bottom. Push the oat mixture firmly into the cavity. You will need to bake the apples a little longer, until they are just tender.

> **THIS RECIPE ALSO MAKES A DELICIOUS BREAKFAST, THAT'S IF YOU CAN RESIST EATING THEM ALL!**

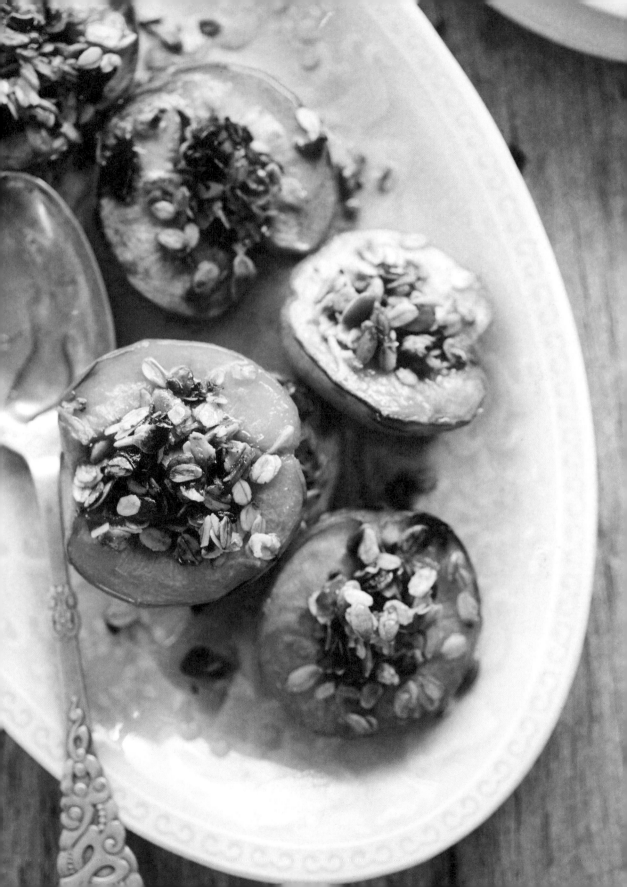

"SOMETIMES IT'S GOOD TO REMIND OURSELVES THAT WE DON'T HAVE TO DO WHAT EVERYONE ELSE IS DOING."

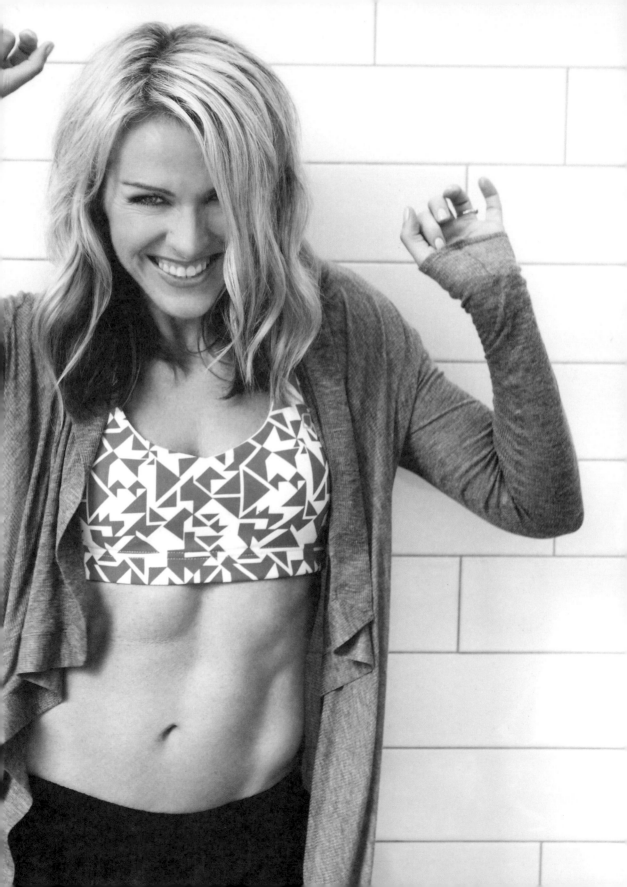

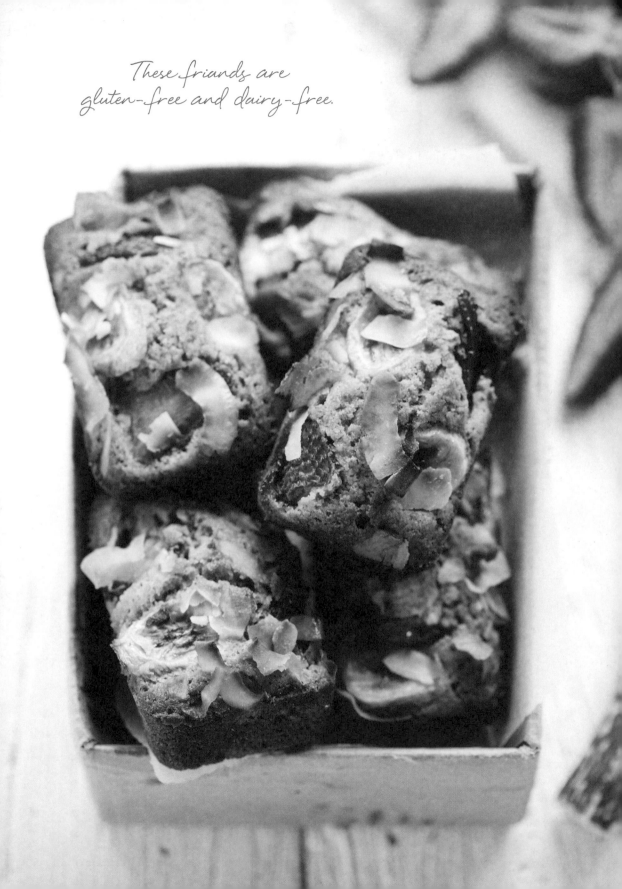

These friands are
gluten-free and dairy-free.

strawberry, banana and almond friands

2 medium bananas (400g)

6 organic free-range egg whites

½ cup (125g) cold-pressed extra-virgin coconut oil

1 cup (120g) ground almonds (meal)

¾ cup (165g) coconut sugar

½ cup (80g) brown rice flour

¼ cup (40g) quinoa flour

1½ teaspoons ground cinnamon

½ teaspoon gluten-free baking powder

4 strawberries, sliced thinly

⅓ cup (15g) flaked coconut or flaked almonds

1 Preheat oven to 200°C/400°F. Grease 8-hole (½-cup/125ml) mini loaf pan; line bases of pan holes with strips of baking paper, extending paper 2.5cm (1-inch) above sides.
2 Thinly slice half of one of the bananas. Mash remaining banana in a small bowl; you will have ½ cup mashed banana.
3 Whisk egg whites in a medium bowl until frothy. Add coconut oil, ground almonds, sugar, mashed banana, sifted flours, cinnamon and baking powder; whisk until combined. Divide mixture evenly into pan holes. Top with sliced banana, strawberries and coconut.
4 Bake friands about 25 minutes. Stand friands in pan for 5 minutes, before transferring onto a wire rack to cool.

prep + cook time 45 minutes **makes** 8
nutritional count per friand protein (8g), carbohydrate (39.6g), total fat (24.5g), fibre (2.6g).

cook's notes

You can use ¾ cup spelt flour, instead of the brown rice flour and quinoa flour, if you prefer, but note the cakes will no longer be gluten free as spelt contains a low amount of gluten.

raw chocolate and chia cake with berries

10 fresh dates (200g), seeded, chopped coarsely

⅔ cup (90g) hazelnuts

⅔ cup (70g) walnuts

⅔ cup (90g) macadamias

⅓ cup (35g) cacao powder

2 tablespoons raw honey

1 teaspoon vanilla bean paste

125g (4 ounces) strawberries, halved

125g (4 ounces) raspberries

125g (4 ounces) blueberries

⅓ cup (15g) flaked coconut

CHOCOLATE CHIA MOUSSE

2½ cups (625ml) coconut cream

½ cup (50g) cacao powder

2 tablespoons raw honey

1½ teaspoons vanilla bean paste

¾ cup (120g) white chia seeds

CHOCOLATE GANACHE

½ cup (125ml) cold-pressed extra-virgin coconut oil

½ cup (50g) cacao powder

1 tablespoon raw honey

1 Grease a 20cm (8-inch) round springform cake pan; line base and side of pan with baking paper.

2 Process dates, nuts, cacao powder, honey and vanilla until well combined. Press mixture into base of pan, smooth surface. Refrigerate 30 minutes.

3 To make chocolate chia mousse, whisk coconut cream, cacao, honey, vanilla and chia seeds in a large jug until combined. Pour mixture into pan over base; refrigerate 3 hours or until firm.

4 To make ganache, whisk coconut oil, cacao powder and honey together in a small bowl. Cover; refrigerate 20 minutes, stirring occasionally, until thickened and spreadable.

5 Remove cake from pan; discard lining papers. Position cake on serving plate or cake stand. Spread ganache over top of cake. Sprinkle with berries and coconut.

prep + cook time 45 minutes (+ refrigeration) **serves** 10
nutritional count per serving protein (10.8g), carbohydrate (34.1g), total fat (48.1g), fibre (8.9g).

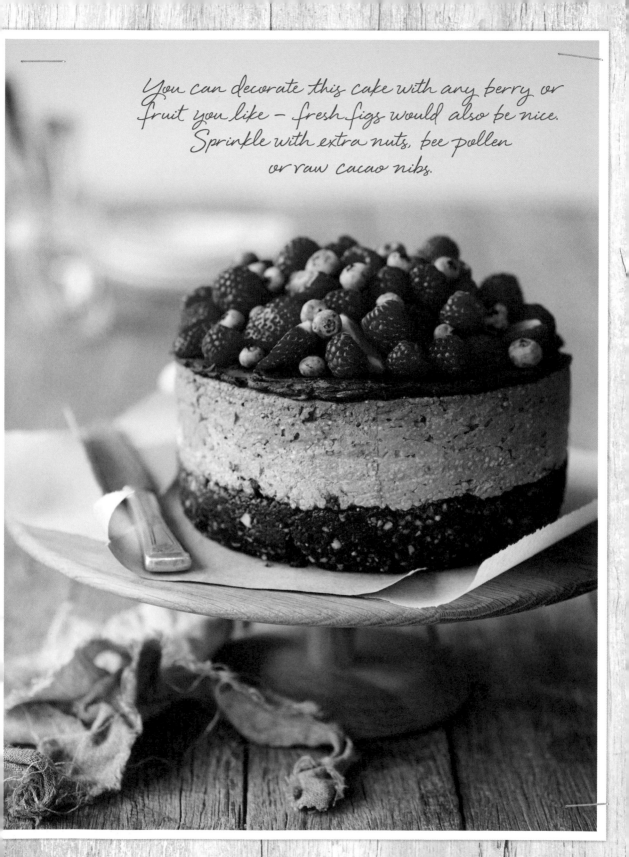

You can decorate this cake with any berry or fruit you like – fresh figs would also be nice. Sprinkle with extra nuts, bee pollen or raw cacao nibs.

HERBAL TEA

I LOVE HERBAL TEAS! NO LONGER THE BREW OF CHOICE ONLY FOR HEALTH FANATICS, THEY ARE CALMING, REVIVING AND HEALING, AND HAVE BECOME MAINSTREAM AS AN INCREASING NUMBER OF PEOPLE DISCOVER THEIR EXOTIC FLAVOURS, MEDICINAL AND SOOTHING QUALITIES.

There are literally hundreds of different blends you can experiment with and I love to draw from them, depending on how I'm feeling on any given day and what time of the day it is.

Here is a guide to some of my favourites:

If you're looking for a vitamin C boost, brew some rosehip tea. It will strengthen your immune system and it also has wonderful anti-ageing properties.

- - - - - - - - - -

For an upset tummy, grate some fresh ginger and infuse it in boiling water for a few minutes, with a squeeze of lemon. I also do this at the first sign of a sore throat and add some manuka honey for its medicinal benefits too.

- - - - - - - - - - - -

SIPPING PEPPERMINT TEA AFTER DINNER FRESHENS YOUR BREATH AND AIDS DIGESTION.

- - -

Chamomile tea is calming and will prepare you for a good night's sleep.

- - - - - - - - - - -

Jasmine tea helps to reduce inflammation and promotes sleep and relaxation. It also has an antibacterial and antiviral effect, so it's good to drink when you feel a cold coming on.

- - - - - - - - - - -

CINNAMON TEA BALANCES BLOOD SUGAR, EASES DIGESTIVE DISCOMFORT AND IS THOUGHT TO BE AN APHRODISIAC!

- - - - - - - - - - -

Spice up your morning ritual of warm lemon water by adding a pinch of cayenne pepper. This combination triggers your digestive system, flushes your liver from its night of detoxing, as well as heals and repairs and alkalises tissues to boost immunity.

- - - - - -

FINALLY, TO ENHANCE THE BENEFITS OF YOUR HERBAL TEA, DISSOLVE A SPOONFUL OF HONEY INTO IT. HONEY IS A CELL FOOD THAT IS READILY ABSORBED, HELPING YOUR BODY TO RECEIVE THE GOODNESS OF THE HERBS – SO ENJOY!

- - - - - - - - -

preparing for change

In a world full of 'busy', food has almost become an inconvenience. We're always complaining that we don't have enough time to eat well and we continually use time as our excuse when we reach for unhealthy options and takeaways. Not anymore. I'm here to show you that with a little foresight and some weekend planning, you can find the time you need to nourish yourself the right way – every day of your life.

Planning ahead is second nature for me, because I'm that girl who takes her food with her wherever she goes. I pack my lunch and snacks for work every day. I take an Esky with me when I fly and there are always snacks, fruit and protein powder in my bag for whenever I might need them.

I understand that preparation is key when it comes to good nutrition. So most Sundays you'll find me in the kitchen getting my food ready for the week ahead. It begins with a little forward thinking about what I will be doing in the week, followed by a big shop at the local farmer's market.

If I have a busy week of meetings, I might start my days with a bigger breakfast than usual and I make sure there are plenty of nutritious snacks on hand in case I don't have time for lunch. I always have a few lunches and dinners in my fridge and some back-up soups and free-range, organic chicken in the freezer.

Salads are easy to prepare ahead of time and will keep up to three days in the fridge. I also make fresh dressings and put them in individual containers that are quick and easy to grab and go. I poach some chicken to slice as I need it and a frittata made on Sunday afternoon can last me up to four days in a sealed container in the fridge.

Snacks are easy and a homemade batch of healthy cookies, breakfast bars or energy balls can be frozen to grab at a minute's notice. The same goes for smoothies – with all the ingredients pre-measured and put into individual freezer bags, they are ready to blend and go as I need them.

There are no strict rules to follow here, except to think about what you have to achieve in the week ahead and then organise your meals and snacks according to what you think your body will need.

I don't advocate counting calories or following strict meal plans, but I have outlined a selection of eating plans for you in the following pages to help you on your way.

The first eating plan is to 'get you started', if being healthy is new for you. The second one is for you to use as a guideline to prepare for a busy high 'energy' week ahead and the third one is to 'cleanse' your body and help you get back on track if you have been travelling or feel your digestive system needs a little rest and recovery.

Planning ahead can be your best friend when it comes to good nutrition. It ensures that you are prepared wherever you go with tasty, nutritious food. And it also guarantees that you won't find yourself hungry with no other options than unhealthy ones.

> ❝ NO GOAL WAS EVER MET WITHOUT A LITTLE PLANNING. ❞

Eating Plan to Get You Started

A balanced meal plan designed to help you eliminate processed foods from your diet and get you started on the road to healthy eating.

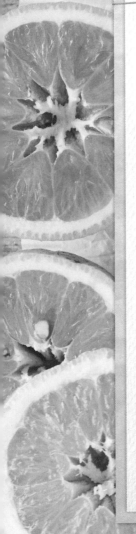

	Monday	Tuesday	Wednesday
Wake-up	Metabolism-Booster Elixir	Beauty Tonic	Immunity Tonic
Breakfast	Roasted Balsamic Tomato and Avocado on Toast	Omelette	Fruit Salad with Passionfruit Yoghurt
Lunch	Frittata	Chicken Sang Choy Bow	Roasted Beetroot and Lentil Salad
Dinner	Tamari, Lime and Sesame Beef and Broccoli Stir-fry	Grilled Miso Salmon with Bean and Pea Salad	Beef Ragu with Zucchini Pasta
Snacks	Ultimate Smoothie	Cacao, Chia and Hazelnut Protein Balls	Ultimate Smoothie
	Chicken and Mung Bean Meatloaf Muffin	Seed Crackers with Lemon and Thyme Carrot Dip	Chicken and Mung Bean Meatloaf Muffin

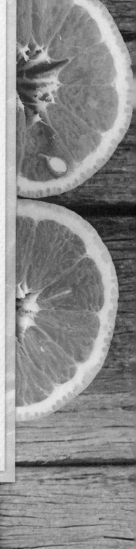

Thursday	Friday	Saturday	Sunday
Metabolism-Booster Elixir	Beauty Tonic	Metabolism-Booster Elixir	Immunity Tonic
Smashed Eggs with Spinach on Toast	Roasted Balsamic Tomato and Avocado on Toast	Omelette	Smashed Eggs with Spinach on Toast
Roasted Pear, Kumara and Brussels Sprout Salad	Lamb and Mint Patties with Pomegranate and Sunflower Sprout Salad	Salmon, Mint and Cucumber Rice Paper Rolls	Chicken Sang Choy Bow
Chilli, Honey and Tamari Fish Bundles with Asian Greens	Chilli, Ginger and Lemon Grass Grilled Chicken with Rainbow Salad	Mustard Beef with Kumara Mash	Spiced Fish with Quinoa Tabouleh and Eggplant Puree
Coconut Yoghurt with Mixed Berries	Ginger Balls	Cottage Cheese and Mixed Berries on Toast	Cacao, Chia and Hazelnut Protein Balls
Seed Crackers with Lemon and Thyme Carrot Dip	Ultimate Smoothie	Seed Crackers with Lemon and Thyme Carrot Dip	Choc-Crunch Banana

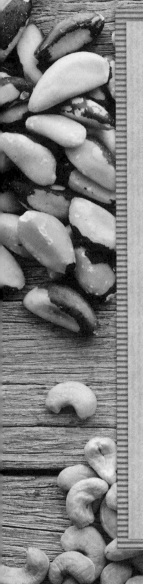

Eating plan for energy

A plan to give you lots of energy. Perfect for those days or weeks when you have a busy schedule and need to be at your very best.

	Monday	Tuesday	Wednesday
Wake-up	Energy Tonic	Happiness Tonic	Energy Tonic
Breakfast	Breakfast Smoothie	Out-the-door Energy Bar	Overnight Oats Parfait with Berries and Yoghurt
Lunch	Kumara and Peanut Butter Soup	Kale, Black Rice and Raspberry Salad	Thai Fish Patties with Kale, Apple and Coconut Slaw
Dinner	Spiced Fish with Quinoa Tabouleh and Eggplant Puree	Mustard Beef with Kumara Mash	Grilled Miso Salmon with Bean and Pea Salad
Snacks	Tamari and Honey Nut Nibbles	Rescue Smoothie	Energy Smoothie
	Avocado with Lemon and Herbs	Vegie Sticks with Nut Butter	Honey and Sesame Spirulina Balls

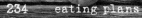

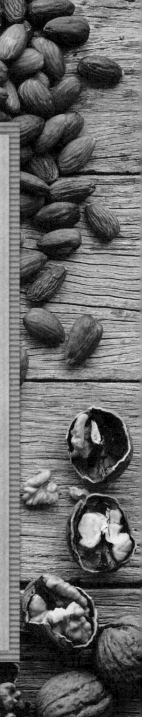

Thursday	Friday	Saturday	Sunday
Happiness Tonic	Energy Tonic	Energy Tonic	Happiness Tonic
Granola with Cinnamon Pears and Coconut Yoghurt	Out-the-door Energy Bar	Corn and Capsicum Fritters with Avocado Salsa	Granola with Cinnamon Pears and Coconut Yoghurt
Mexican Fish and Quinoa Salad	Kumara and Peanut Butter Soup	Lamb and Mint Patties with Pomegranate and Sunflower Sprout Salad	Frittata
Chilli, Ginger and Lemon Grass Grilled Chicken with Rainbow Salad	Seafood Paella	Chilli and Garlic Prawn Skewers with Quinoa and Cauliflower Pilaf	Chilli, Honey and Tamari Fish Bundles with Aisan Greens
Vegie Sticks with Nut Butter	Avocado with Lemon and Herbs	Energy Smoothie	Rescue Smoothie
Tamari and Honey Nut Nibbles	Honey and Sesame Spirulina Balls	Seed Crackers with Lemon and Thyme Carrot Dip	Spinach Hummus with Vegie Sticks

EATING PLAN TO CLEANSE

A meat-free, minimal dairy plan, designed for a short-term detox period.

	Monday	Tuesday	Wednesday
Wake-up	Detox Elixir	Cleanse Elixir	Glow Elixir
Breakfast	Nourishing Breakfast Salad	Fruit Salad with Passionfruit Yoghurt	Overnight Oats Parfait with Berries and Yoghurt
Lunch	Curried Red Lentil Soup	Thai-style Vegetable Rolls	Detox Green Soup
Dinner	Vegetarian Lasagne with Shaved Fennel Salad	Detox Green Soup	Quinoa and Cauliflower Pilaf
Snacks	Wonder Woman Smoothie	Green Smoothie (3 or 4)	Wonder Woman Smoothie
	Spinach Hummus with Vegie Sticks	Caraway Beetroot Dip with Vegie Sticks	Avocado with Lemon and Herbs

Thursday	Friday	Saturday	Sunday
Detox Elixir	Cleanse Elixir	Glow Elixir	Cleanse Elixir
Fruit Salad with Passionfruit Yoghurt	Nourishing Breakfast Salad	Corn and Capsicum Fritters with Avocado Salsa	Nourishing Breakfast Salad
Thai-style Vegetable Rolls	Curried Red Lentil Soup	Detox Green Soup	Roasted Beetroot and Lentil Salad
Roasted Pumpkin, Beetroot, Chickpea and Barley Salad	Vegetarian Lasagne with Shaved Fennel Salad	Quinoa and Cauliflower Pilaf	Quinoa Tabouleh
Green Smoothie (3 or 4)	Green Smoothie (3 or 4)	Wonder Woman Smoothie	Green Smoothie (3 or 4)
Caraway Beetroot Dip with Vegie Sticks	Frozen Grapes or Raspberries	Spinach Hummus with Vegie Sticks	Frozen Grapes or Raspberries

20
healthy habits every woman should have

1. START AFRESH every single day

2. BE HONEST with yourself
and those around you

3. Have your OWN OPINIONS

4. COOK

5. Remember what's right for someone else might
not be what's right for you (and that's okay)

6. Listen to your body

7. PUT DOWN YOUR PHONE
when you're out with people

8. USE SPF and wear a hat in the sun

9. STAND UP FOR YOURSELF

10. Never touch anything
with half your heart

11. Don't skimp on sleep

12. COUNT TO TEN when you're angry

13. Understand that exercise doesn't always have to be a big-time commitment

14. Spend TIME ALONE

15. Never feel embarrassed to LAUGH, CRY, SING or LOVE

16. Consider drinking chlorophyll

17. Believe in HAPPY ENDINGS

18. Read labels on everything from food to make-up

19. Never be afraid to ask for help

20. Live with PASSION

basic recipes

MNB SEED AND NUT BREAD

1 cup (200g) pepitas (pumpkin seeds)

½ cup (75g) sunflower seed kernels

2 tablespoons sesame seeds

2 tablespoons black chia seeds

1 cup (90g) rolled oats

¾ cup (60g) quinoa flakes

1 cup (160g) almond kernels

½ cup (50g) walnuts

1 teaspoon Himalayian rock salt

1¾ cups (430ml) warm filtered water

2 tablespoons cold-pressed
extra-virgin coconut oil

1 tablespoon honey

1 tablespoon each pepitas (pumpkin seeds),
sunflower seed kernels and black chia seeds

1 Grease and line 14cm x 23cm (5½-inch x 9¼-inch) loaf pan with baking paper, extending paper 5cm over long sides.
2 Process seeds, oats, quinoa, nuts and salt until coarsely chopped. Add the water, oil and honey; process mixture until just combined. Spread mixture into pan; sprinkle with extra seeds, press down gently. Cover loosely; stand at room temperature for three hours or overnight. (Loaf will hold its shape when you pull the paper away from the side of the pan.)
3 Preheat oven to 180°C/350°F.
4 Bake bread about 1 hour or until bread sounds hollow when tapped with fingers. Cool bread in pan before slicing.

prep + cook time 1 hour 15 minutes (+standing & cooling) **makes** 16
nutritional count per slice protein (10.6g), carbohydrate (9.1g), total fat (18.9g), fibre (1.9g).

cook's notes

Keep bread, covered, in the fridge for 3-4 days or freeze slices, wrapped tightly in foil or plastic wrap, for up to 3 months.

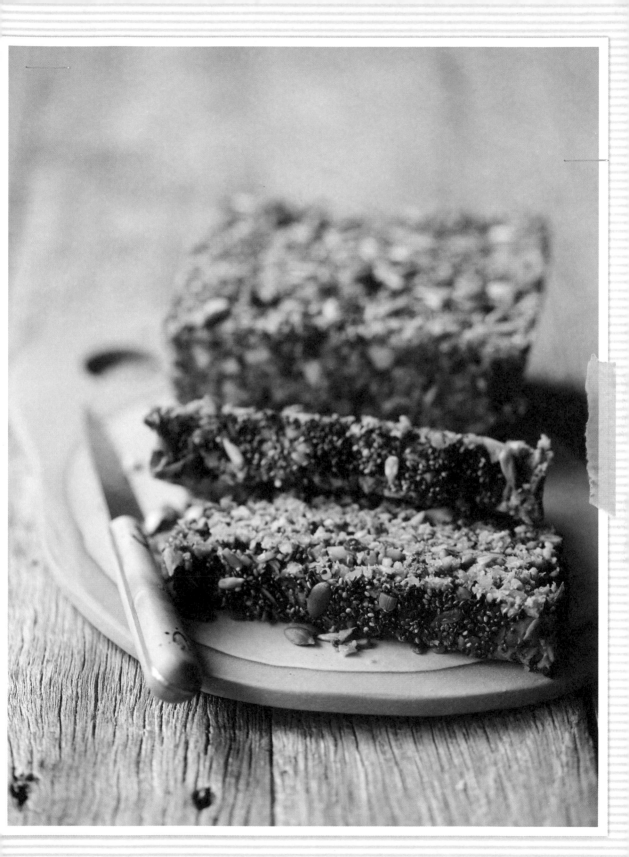

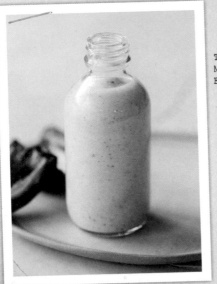

TRY USING THE MACADAMIA
MYLK IN THE BALANCE
ELIXIR RECIPE PAGE 51

coconut mylk

1 fresh young drinking coconut

---

1 Pour coconut water into blender. Using a spoon, scoop out the jelly-like flesh from coconut, add to blender. Blend coconut water and flesh until smooth.

---

prep time 5 minutes
makes 2 cups (500ml)
nutritional count per serving per 1 cup (250ml) protein (0.9g), carbohydrate (12.5g), total fat (2.1g), fibre (0.2g).

macadamia mylk

1 cup (200g) raw macadamias

---

3 cups (750ml) water

---

1 Combine nuts and the water in a medium bowl. Cover; stand at room temperature 3 hours.
2 Blend macadamia mixture until smooth.

---

prep time 5 minutes (+ standing)
makes 1 litre (4 cups)
nutritional count per 1 cup (250ml) protein (3.8g), carbohydrate (2.3g), total fat (38.1g), fibre (3g).

cook's notes

Store macadamia mylk in a sealed glass bottle or jar, in the fridge for 3-4 days. Mixture will separate on standing, shake well before use. You can use any nuts you like. You can also add sweeteners such as vanilla bean paste, pure maple syrup, raw honey or ground cinnamon.

What I love about these mylks is that they don't need to be strained – so take no time at all.

COCONUT MYLK

MACADAMIA MYLK

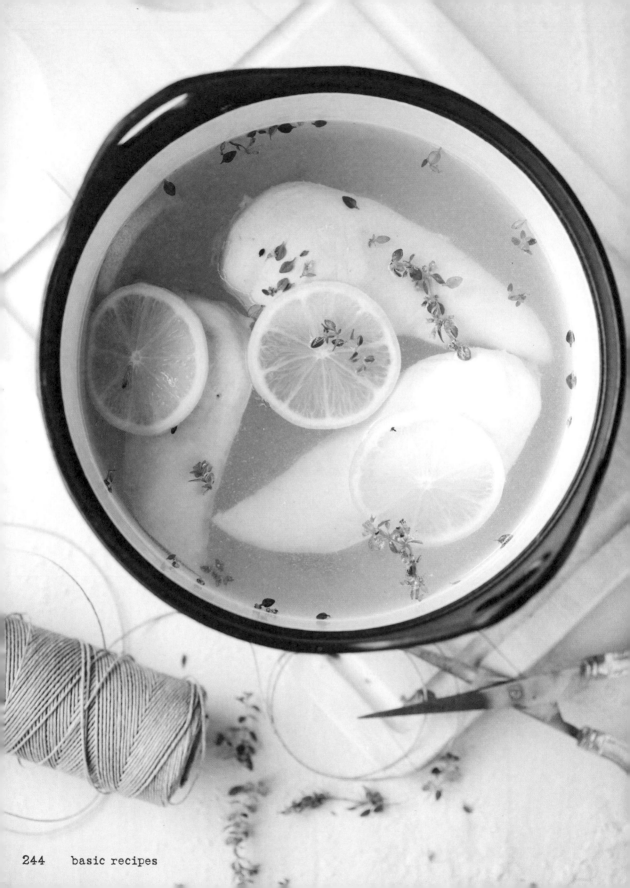

poached chicken

1 chicken breast fillet (200g)
---
1 sprig fresh thyme

½ lemon, sliced
---
3 black peppercorns
---

1 Place all ingredients in a small saucepan; cover with cold water. Bring to the boil. Reduce heat; simmer, covered, 10 minutes. Remove from heat; stand, covered, 10 minutes. Slice or shred chicken meat as desired. Discard poaching liquid. May be frozen.

---

prep + cook time 15 minutes (+ standing)
makes 1 cup shredded chicken
nutritional count per 1 cup protein (44.6g), carbohydrate (0g), total fat (3.2g), fibre (0g).

I always have poached chicken in my fridge — ready to add to salads, soups and frittatas.

Thanks!

To all the super amazing people in my life that not only helped make this book happen, but who are always there to encourage, motivate, support and inspire me every day.

Sending a ton of love and heartfelt appreciation to you all.

Lorna Jane x

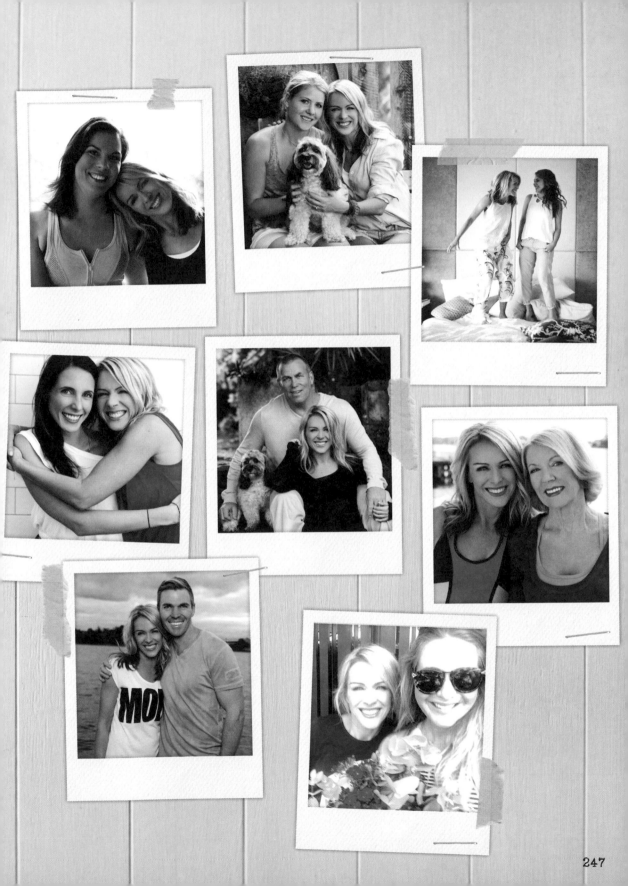

glossary of ingredients

Acai: pronounced 'ah-sigh-EE', a small, round fruit with a hard, inedible pit and a dark purple, pulpy skin that tastes like a blend of berries and chocolate. Available at health food stores or online.

Bee pollen: is pollen produced by flowers that the honeybee returns to the hive. Bee pollen is the main source of nutrient for the bees and their only source of protein. It can be sprinkled on cereal or fruit or added to smoothies. Available in capsule or powder form, at health food stores or online.

Black rice: black rice is also known as 'forbidden rice' and is used throughout Asia in both sweet and savoury dishes. Available at major supermarkets and health food stores.

Brown rice protein powder: is a non-dairy protein extracted from whole grain brown rice that is high in protein and low in fat and carbohydrates. Available at health food stores and online.

Cacao powder: a raw form of cocoa powder which is made by grinding cacao beans and pressing out the cocoa butter (fat). This powder gives an intense chocolate taste to sweet treats. Available at major supermarkets and health food stores.

Cacao butter: the fat extracted from the cacao bean. Cacao is traditionally used to make chocolate. It has a cocoa taste and a rich, velvety texture. It can be found in health food stores.

Chia seeds: seeds from a mint-like plant that is native to South America. Chia seeds have up to eight times more omega-3 than salmon. The seeds come in two colours – black and white – and their nutritional content is identical. Available at major supermarkets, health food stores and online.

Coconut milk: the diluted liquid of the white flesh of a brown coconut from the second pressing (the first richer pressing produces coconut cream). Available at supermarkets.

Cold-pressed extra virgin coconut oil: the oil extracted from the first pressing of the coconut flesh. Available at health food stores and online.

Goji berries: used medicinally in China for centuries. Now grown in Australia and elsewhere, these dried, small, very juicy, sweet red berries are believed to be high in nutrients and antioxidants. Available at supermarkets and health food stores.

Himalayan pink rock salt: an ancient natural rock salt with a rich mineral content. Available at major supermarkets, health food stores and online.

Maca powder: the dried and ground root of the maca plant, also known as 'Peruvian ginseng'. Available at health food stores and online.

Manuka honey: a pure form of honey. Available at supermarkets and health food stores.

Mylk: a medieval spelling of milk, the word is used in this book to describe non-dairy milk products.

Nut butter: peanut butter has long been a pantry staple, but now you can find it made with other nuts. Available at major supermarkets and health food stores.

Patty pan squash: a mild-flavoured squash that looks like a wrinkled, pale green pear. If unavailable, you can use another variety of squash or zucchini.

Pearl barley: a nutritious grain with a mild, nutty flavour. Commonly used in soups, it may also be served cold in salads. Available at supermarkets and health food stores.

Quinoa: pronounced 'keen-wa', this ancient seed can be used in a similar way to grains like couscous or rice. Quinoa flour can be used in gluten-free baking. Quinoa is generally grown organically as the plant naturally provides its own pesticide – saponi – which can taste bitter if the quinoa isn't rinsed thoroughly before using. Available at major supermarkets and health food stores.

Saffron threads: a spice related to the crocus family that is available ground or in strands. Available at most major supermarkets.

Spirulina: a protein-rich algae sold in either tablet or powder form. Available at health food stores or online.

Stevia: a sugar substitute derived from the leaves of the stevia plant that is significantly sweeter than sugar but contains no calories. Available in liquid or powder form at health food stores and online.

Tahini: a Middle-Eastern paste made from sesame seeds and olive oil. Available at supermarkets.

Tamari: a dark, rich Japanese soy sauce. Available at supermarkets and health food stores.

Vanilla bean paste: made from the scraped-out vanilla pod. Vanilla bean paste is highly concentrated and available at major supermarkets.

CONVERSION CHART

MEASURES

One Australian metric measuring cup holds approximately 250ml; one Australian metric tablespoon holds 20ml; one Australian metric teaspoon holds 5ml.

The difference between one country's measuring cups and another's is within a two- or three-teaspoon variance, and will not affect your cooking results. North America, New Zealand and the United Kingdom use a 15ml tablespoon.

All cup and spoon measurements are level. The most accurate way of measuring dry ingredients is to weigh them. When measuring liquids, use a clear glass or plastic jug with the metric markings.

The imperial measurements used in these recipes are approximate only. Measurements for cake pans are approximate only. Using same-shaped cake pans of a similar size should not affect the outcome of your baking. We measure the inside top of the cake pan to determine sizes.

We used large eggs with an average weight of 60g.

LENGTH MEASURES

METRIC	IMPERIAL
3mm	⅛in
6mm	¼in
1cm	½in
2cm	¾in
2.5cm	1in
5cm	2in
6cm	2½in
8cm	3in
10cm	4in
13cm	5in
15cm	6in
18cm	7in
20cm	8in
22cm	9in
25cm	10in
28cm	11in
30cm	12in (1ft)

LIQUID MEASURES

METRIC	IMPERIAL
30ml	1 fluid oz
60ml	2 fluid oz
100ml	3 fluid oz
125ml	4 fluid oz
150ml	5 fluid oz
190ml	6 fluid oz
250ml	8 fluid oz
300ml	10 fluid oz
500ml	16 fluid oz
600ml	20 fluid oz
1000ml (1 litre)	1¾ pints

DRY MEASURES

METRIC	IMPERIAL
15g	½oz
30g	1oz
60g	2oz
90g	3oz
125g	4oz (¼lb)
155g	5oz
185g	6oz
220g	7oz
250g	8oz (½lb)
280g	9oz
315g	10oz
345g	11oz
375g	12oz (¾lb)
410g	13oz
440g	14oz
470g	15oz
500g	16oz (1lb)
750g	24oz (1½lb)
1kg	32oz (2lb)

OVEN TEMPERATURES

The oven temperatures in this book are for conventional ovens; if you have a fan-forced oven, decrease the temperature by 10-20 degrees.

	°C (CELSIUS)	°F (FAHRENHEIT)
Very slow	120	250
Slow	150	300
Moderately slow	160	325
Moderate	180	350
Moderately hot	200	400
Hot	220	425
Very hot	240	475

RECIPE INDEX

Published by Lorna Jane.
Designed and printed by Bauer Media Books.

Author: Lorna Jane Clarkson
Creative Designer: Tara McCafferty
Design: Hieu Nguyen
Food Editor: Rhiannon Mack
Food Photographer: Cath Muscat
Food Stylist: Sarah O'Brien
Lifestyle photographer: Jason Zambelli
Photochef: Arum Shim
Printed in China.

National Library of Australia Cataloguing-in-Publication entry:
Author: Clarkson, Lorna Jane
Title: Nourish : the fit woman's cookbook / Lorna Jane Clarkson.
ISBN: 9780646920825 (pbk.)
Subjects: Cooking. Nutrition.
Dewey Number: 641.563

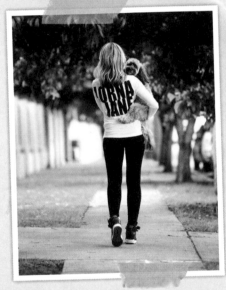

While all care has been taken in researching and compiling the dietary
information in this book, all opinions in this book are those of the author only
and are not a substitute for any medical treatment. If you suspect you have a
medical problem you are advised to seek professional medical help. Readers
are advised to check with their medical professional before relying on or
otherwise making use of the dietary information in this book.